## Preface

I was sitting down and realizing how blessed I am able to eat and sleep well. Money can never buy it. I want to share with everyone how simple changes in life style can improve our health.

## Acknowledgement

Special thanks to Mr. Bradshaw for giving me advice about exercise.

# Success Stories

## Jennifer Weeks

When I started my weight loss journey, I mentioned to Dr. Fazal, he counseled me on his plan with which he experienced great success. I was positively alarmed at his transformation and his results motivated me to engage. Initially, I was skeptical as it seemed easy and too good to be true. I decided to give it a try and encountered great success! I found the plan easy to maintain with lots of choices and not starving myself. I lost a total of 50lbs and the weight has stayed off! Bottom line up front, it's all about knowing what you can and cannot eat and how various foods impact your body's functioning. I highly recommend this plan to anyone considering losing weight or desiring to develop healthy eating practices. It works!

# Carl Guthrie, 46years

After being very athletic and serving in the military for 10 years leg injuries, which made it difficult and painful to walk or run, caused me to stop exercising at all. Over the next 10 years, I slowly gained 70lbs which resulted in high blood pressure and elevated cholesterol levels.  I was prescribed medication for the high blood pressure and stayed on this medication for 5 years but what really concerned me was when my doctor, at a yearly physical, told me I had developed pre-diabetes.  If I didn't get my A1C down I would be put on insulin and this is usually a one way trip, meaning once I started taking insulin my body would probably stop producing it and I would be on it for the rest of my life. This was my wake up call, and I heard it loud and clear!

As a result I changed my diet, I still eat just about everything, but I control the portions and where healthier alternatives exist, try to use them to reduce carbohydrates and sugar.

I also start incorporating physical exercise in the form of walking. At first I just started walking for 30 minutes, slowly increasing the time I would walk and my speed. I'm now walking 4 to 6 miles a day 6 days each week, and I have lost 56 lbs.  I'm no longer taking any medication to control my blood pressure and my A1C is back at normal levels.

Today I have formulated eating habits that are easy for me to continue, as a matter a fact I eat more than I did before, choosing healthier options in controlled portions, spaced at 3-4-hour intervals. The biggest change is that I take at least one hour a day for a walk or exercise of some type no matter what. I feel so much better, and my energy is tenfold what it was before the weight loss.

Medical Disclaimer. ... The Content is not intended to be a substitute for professional medical advice, diagnosis, or treatment. Always seek the advice of your physician or other qualified health provider with any questions you may have regarding a medical condition.

To my parents Aami, Abuji

For their prayers, they taught me to pursue my dreams and serve humanity and spread message of love no matter what

Siblings Faheem, Kaleem, Salman,Hamad, Rehan, Amna, Aasia Smiling from Heaven Numan, Adila

Part of our loving family

My love my better half Farah
Always standing by me and wind beneath my wings

If you cannot explain it simply, then you don't understand it well enough

Albert Einstein

# Contents

We experience miracles every day, we are blessed every morning when we wake up, that we can move our bodies, look at our love ones and be thankful that we are alive. There are many in this world who have everything but health. I would like to share with the world just how I realized this and began to appreciate the blessing we have.

Diet plays important role in all aspects of life, as its one of our most basic of instincts, we work hard so we can eat. Every generation has ventured out to find good food when they felt hungry, our ancestors, even when living in caves, went out to hunt. There are lot of books about food, diet and weight loss available, and I am not saying anything which you do not already know, but I feel I can tell you in the simplest, easy to understand way. I feel that being as this is an issue that affects us all, I am compelled to share how I accomplished my goals. I did not spend money. I just made the right choices.

Like everyone, I struggled with weight and associated health issues. My struggle had been going on for a long time, but it never really occurred to me that it was so simple to deal with, until I understood health is the real wealth.

The answer is simple, but I had to realize it for myself. It was always there, but I could never see that solution was right in front of me, I just needed the vision to see it. We sleep and wake up every day, but don't take time to appreciate our time, our lives, our blessings, and more importantly our health.

We are blessed with all of these things, but we need to take care of our bodies to keep enjoying our life and count our blessings. It is important to enjoy life and diet. My current diet is I can continue forever as this is my first and last step.

## Last step first

It is important to figure out the final destination, where you want to be at the end, because if you are going to set that goal, you would more likely lose weight and keep it off. So, live that life, lose the weight and enjoy your health.

When I went to dietitian for the first time, I found it very difficult to eat any preserved foods. I told my wife it will be impossible to diet. Interestingly, since I purchased packages I never used them. I threw them after 7 months.

I started to realize more that any diet effort is life style change and not one-month trial.

## Wrong Habits

There was a time I would just look for food, we would go out and eat every day. I would try every cuisine, Thai, Asian, American, Vietnam, Chinese, Indian, Mediterranean and so forth. I even learnt to fly so I could eat in my favorite restaurants in Chicago. I would fly 2hrs just to eat. I was delighted to eat carbohydrates and try all kind of foods, it did not matter if I was happy or sad. I would sometimes eat more if I were sad, and sometimes less, but I would still eat, like most people. Eating became the only form of reward I had for myself. the question was, how did it start, and where did I change, where did I wrong?

I was so skinny in medical school at age 22, It was easy to fast and eat, and I never had headaches, high blood pressure or an urge to keep eating. Why were things suddenly different, and what was causing it?

1.Social Norms

The big question about my situation was how I learned to gain weight. I remember when I was seeing patients during my medical school years, I had a few patients who saw me as a doctor while I was learning as a medical student, during my training years. One patient asked me where the doctor was, and I said I'm your doctor or student doctor, he joked with me, saying "You are so lightweight that you cannot possibly be a doctor, doctors always seemed to be much bigger guys!". It was at that time unfortunately the culture was also the same, encouraging physicians and professionals to look heavy. I wanted to do things to please others at the expense of my own health.

One of my friends once told me they tried to lose weight in Alaska, and within a few weeks everyone started asking if they were sick. Hard to understand but we expect men to be big size. No wonder average men die earlier than women.

## 2.Portion Increases

I decided that I was going to eat a lot, so I started eating large quantities of rice and quickly gained weight, I gained 5 pounds and some belly fat. I talked with my friends and they were impressed that I could gain weight finally. I felt more confident, I looked as people expected, that I had graduated and was a doctor now. I could see people and not feel ashamed that I was so lightweight. So, I tried to do things which I was not originally made to do. and then to please others I tried to gain weight and to look heavier. I succeeded, and over the years my family kept telling me to lose weight, but I wanted to look professional and look great in front of others.

Eventually I developed kidney stones, and I had lab tests done which showed my sugar levels were high. I checked my HgbA1C, which measures your 3 month average sugar levels, and my hemoglobin A-1 C jumped from normal to 6.1. At the same time I started to develop some infections, especially fungal infections around my toes. To deal with this I decided to walk every day, which I did. 30 minutes every day, then after three months I checked my A-1 C. It was 6.3, and realizing this was a problem, I started to do some exercise. After a short time though, I gave up my exercise, and one year later I checked my blood work, which showed my A-1 C had climbed again, this time to 6.4.

I knew that I had a real problem and checked with my doctor. He gave me two options, the first was to do diet and exercise aggressively, the second to start on medications. I was confident that I could do this through exercise, because I did not want to use the medication. I had read about the medications, including metformin, and it worried me. I constantly checked for G.I. symptoms, glipizide, medication, checking sugar so frequently I was almost trying to will a result, I knew that I needed to walk my sugar down, and if I didn't, then it would go up further, even as far as the 140s.

## Stepping Stone

When change comes, it is often following a close call, and I had one. It happened to me one day when I was driving, just enjoying music in my car and watching the world go by. My pulse became irregular, I was worried by this, so I pulled over. I never passed out, but my vision was distorted, it's difficult to describe, but it was like everything changed from a 3-dimensional image to a 2 dimensional one. Then concentric dark circles started, first in my peripheral vision then they narrowed, appearing as a dark tunnel with no end in sight. I finally saw light, and to this day I thank God nothing happened. I was back to my life, but thinking more and appreciatively of the blessings I have.

I went to see my health care provider the very next day, taking cardiology tests and CT scans. Luckily, my arteries were clear, and the cardiologist suggested weight loss. That is when I realized that maybe I should try, at least once.

The next day made an appointment to see a dietitian, she was very helpful, and we went over my goals, my target weight and she gave me some guidance about protein carbohydrates and fats within my diet. I looked at the diet program she created, but I felt it was not for me. It was hard to imagine myself leaving pancakes, bread, pasta and deserts out of my diet at that point.

However, I thought I should try at least once. But not the diet I have been given, the food tasted so bad that it just made me want to give up instead of keep trying.

Instead, I thought that I could try to think about the concepts of a diet, I had medical knowledge and now was the time to put it into practice. I tried to remember what was at stake. I was at crossroads, the choice was either to take medications for the rest of my life or make changes to my life style. I just recalled that moment, how it felt, as I was just passing through that black tunnel. It was blessing that I saw light again, and knew that I could find a way to make the diet work.

I studied the basic concepts of diet again and tried to keep things simple, just deal with basic facts.

## Disease connections

## Headaches

I used to feel hungry and crave food soon after eating.  I would get headaches.

## Hypertension

My blood pressure started to rise into the 130's range and remain there. I started to do some regular walking, and this helped a little, but again after a while my levels got worse.

I began to snore really badly as well. I had a home study done, looking at my Apnea Hypopnea Index AHI which measures quiet breathing Apnea or hypopnea partial quiet breathing was less than 5, but REM (Rapid Eye Movement) or Dream AHI was high. This was something else I was hoping to improve.

Even trying everything, all the diets, all the exercise, I never lost weight for so many months it.

I came up with simple plan, and it worked! So, I would like to share with everyone, if I can help just one person, it will all be worthwhile.

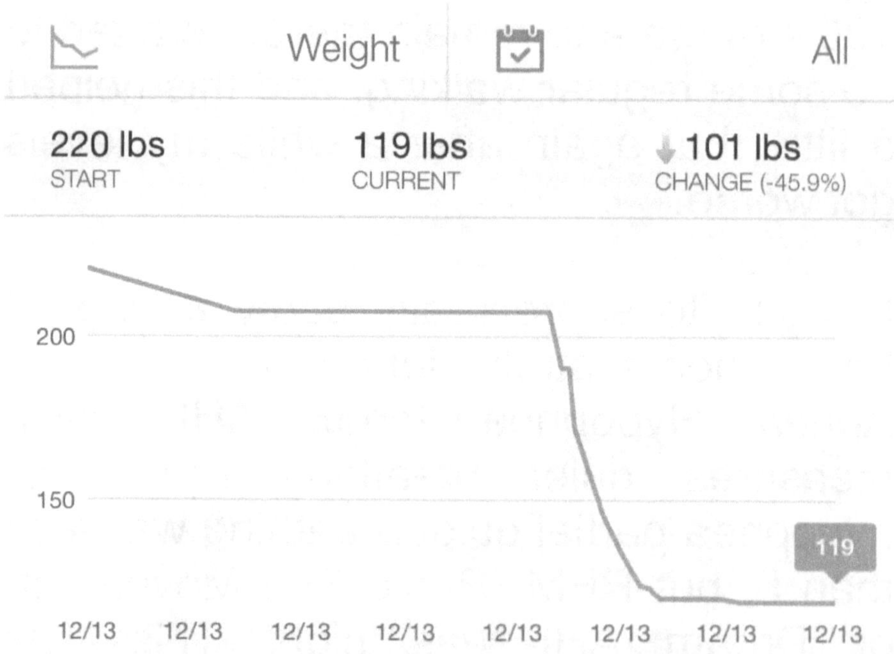


1/2016 till 12/2018

# My hard work paid off

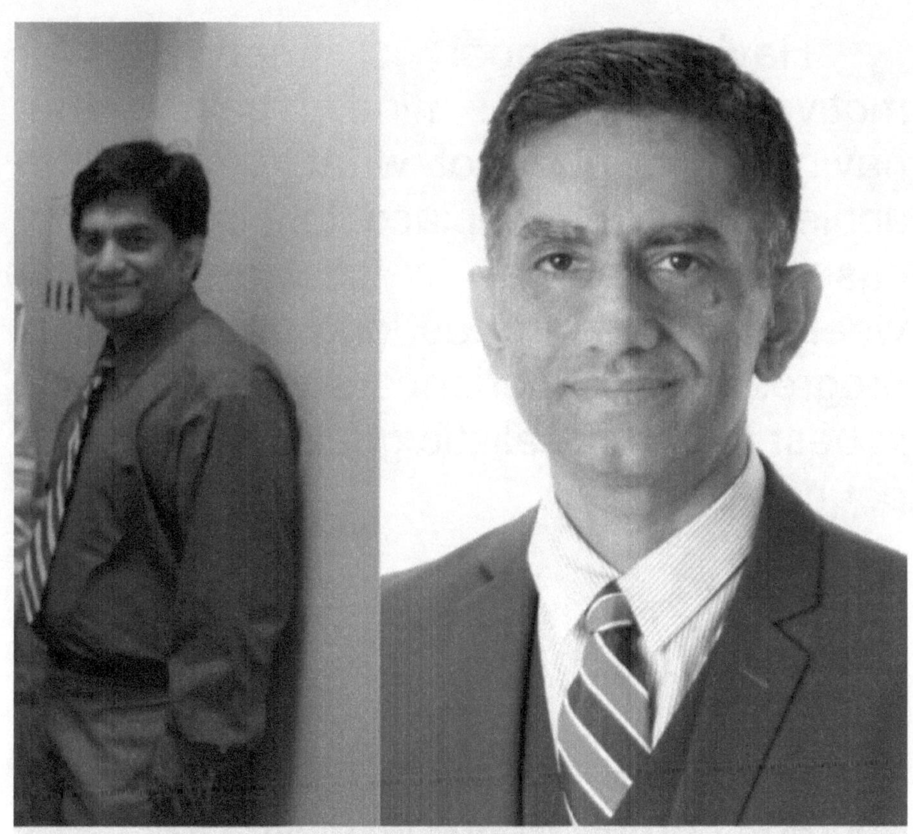

**Back to life**

**Define Goals**

Having a goal is important for motivation, so I set mine. I believe that having some idea of what we need to achieve is a good place to start. In my case, the goal was to lose weight in 4 weeks, any amount as long as there was progress. My experience suggests that it is best to have realistic goals, like 0.5 to 1 pounds per week.

**Baby Steps**

Eliminate carbohydrate percentage and add complex carbohydrates

Add protein over the next 3 days, I ate eggs and chicken, along with some bread and lettuce.

Over the next week I crossed a major land mark, my weight dipped below 205 for the first time in over year. I realized that I had lost 3 lbs in just one week! Even then, I did not follow the diet completely all the time.

My fasting blood sugar level was 100, and post meal was 120 and that was without any medications.

I bought a treadmill, like so many people have done before, and had made yearly promises to lose weight, again like so many others, but as many do, I always gave up in a few weeks. Last year I bought 3 more machines, an Ab cruncher, and elliptical exerciser and a rowing machine. I played racquetball, had all types of apps, fitness memberships, everything, but I never lost any weight until I tried this.

For me the fasting month was so hard, I would get terrible headaches. It was so hard to work after breaking fast but now everything was easy.

Nothing feels better than success, even if it's just a few pounds.

Let's get on with it and look at the basics

## <u>Basic Concepts</u>

First, let us look at just how we can measure our health when it comes to weight related issues, there are several factors to look at.

Metabolism:

This is the BMI, or basal metabolic index, for ages above 20 and if you are if not pregnant, calculated by height/weight. It is the same for men and women.
**Formula: Weight in lbs x703/ inch Sq Height**

WHO Classification:

| BMI Value | Classification |
|---|---|
| Less than 18.5 | Underweight |

| 18.5 – 24.9 | Normal Weight |
| 25 – 29.9 | Overweight |
| 30 – 34.9 | Type I Obese |
| 35 – 39.9 | Type II Obese |
| 40 – 44.9 | Type III Obese |

Remember it can overestimate your BMI if you have a muscular build, and underestimate it if you are low on muscle mass.

Waist ratio is important, for non-Asians in the USA, men's waist measurements above 40 inches means health risks, For Asian men, 36 inches is the level that risk becomes a factor. For USA Women a waist measurement of 36 inches or higher is a risk, and for Asian women 32inches or higher is risk factor. Other ethnic populations have different figures.

Obesity is often more related to medical complications such as Diabetes 2, Heart disease or Metabolic syndrome. Hip to waist ratio, which we get by dividing hip measured at the trochanteric area and waist above the Iliac crest, for men a value over 0.9 and for women a ratio over 0.85 is important.

Body Fat Percentage, which we get by calculating the total body fat as percentage of total body weight.

Here is the formula:

Body Fat percentage= 1.2 x BMI + 0.23 x age - 5.4 – 10.8 x Gender (Female 0, Male 1)

I use over 25 percent for Men for Obesity, 30 % for women

BMR or Basal metabolic rate, is amount in calories that we need to function at rest, we need to calculate average needs daily based on activity and weight, calculated by formula, Certain factors affect it some are age, activity, sex, muscle mass. Lean body mass.

For Men,
BMR= 10 x wt. in kg + 6.25 x Ht. in cm -5 age in yrs+5

For Women,
BMR=10 x wt. in kg + 6.25 x Ht. in cm -5 age in yrs-161

BMR can also be adjusted for activity

For BMR, calories are used for vital organs, functioning and processes. How many calories can vary from person to person, and ranges from 1200 to 2300 per day. Some of factors include activity and the person's fat free mass.

BMR can be affected by muscle mass, however activity is even more important.

Fats are used to store energy within the body.

Carbohydrates are a rapid supply fuel, and can be changed into anything the body needs, and can be used by the brain and muscles without insulin.

Proteins in muscle produces 9 kcal of heat. Protein is present in animal meats, and has 2/3 proteins and 1/3 carbohydrates present. There is also protein in lentils, they have 1/3 protein and 2/3 carbohydrates.

Now, let's go over some basic concepts of the mechanics of eating itself. When we chew food, it is basically crushed by the mouth and teeth and it is swallowed down the esophagus into the stomach area. Once here, the stomach area receives messages from the brain that food is coming, triggering the digestive process to absorb the nutrients. This starts in the small intestine where the digestion begins, and then carries on through the first part of the small intestine, the duodenum, then the most effective digestive process, which occurs in the small intestine, the ileum, and then the waste food is passed on to the large intestine, where a stool is formed and excreted. The liver is the most important organ in the digestive process, as it excretes bile, while also metabolizing and storing nutrients and vitamins.

The pancreas secretes insulin and glucagon, hormones which lower or increase blood sugars.

Let us look at brain, we have specific portions of brain doing important functions.

Let us look at the brain, there are specific portions of the brain doing various important functions.

We have a hunger center, which is the Lateral Hypothalamus part of the Limbic portion, or primitive brain (which controls sex, food, thirst, emotions).

We have the Satiety Center which tells us to stop eating, found in the Venteromedial Hypothalmus.

We have the Reward Center, which is found in the Striatum area, also called the Lateral hypothalamus. The Ventromedial nuclei area mainly secretes Dopamine.

Our hunger center is present in the hypothalamus portion of the brain, and if the stomach has insufficient food it secretes hormones such as Grehlin.

The satiety center does the opposite of the hunger center, if enough food is present, the hormone Leptin inhibits hunger via the satiety center.

The brain controls all of this by using hormones as well as nerves, especially the Vagus nerve, which is present in the stomach and other areas of the body.

Nerves, especially in the upper part of the stomach, send information to the brain from areas of the stomach which can basically give us that full feeling, telling us we're done eating.

The body breaks up energy from Carbohydrates, fats and proteins to provide energy using a process known as Catabolism or breakdown. It can also build by a process called Anabolism, seen in bodily operations such as building muscle.

At rest or in Aerobic state, more energy derived from fats than Carbohydrates is used by the body.

With exercise, more carbohydrates are used, and if the exercise is intense, mostly carbohydrates are consumed.

<u>Remember Grehlin Grows Hunger, Leptin Lowers it.</u>

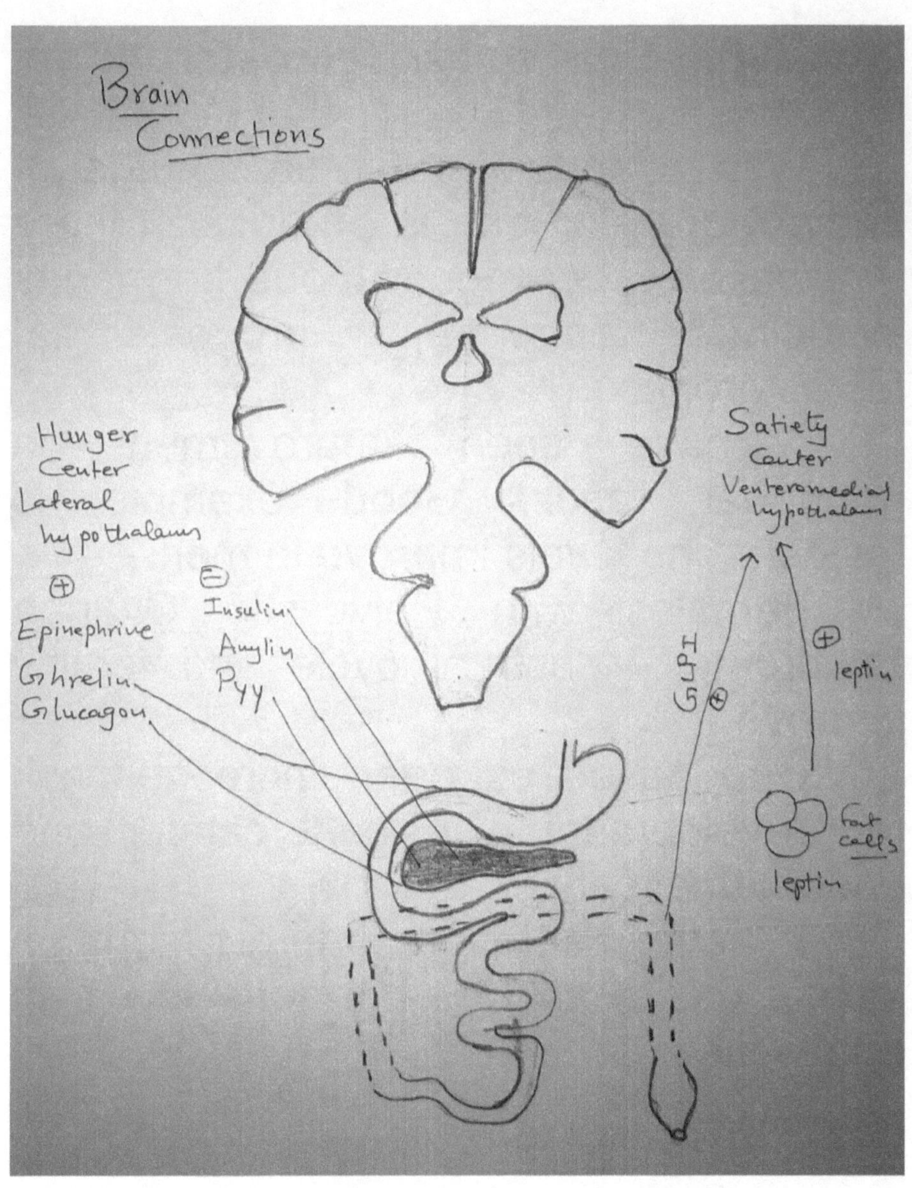


# Hunger Center/ Satiety Center

# Improving Hormones/ Testosterone

With changes in fat percentage of body, more estrogen is produced. There is a balance between various hormones including estrogen, progesterone, testosterone.

I have seen improvement in hormonal ratios. Good example is testosterone levels improve in men.

Females with Polycystic Ovarian Syndrome, Menstrual cycle and fertility improve.

Unopposed estrogen increases risk for development of Breast cancer and endometrial cancer.

I have seen an improvement in sexual desire as well hormone levels in both sexes.

**Glucose story**

After food is absorbed it causes insulin to be released, especially when carbohydrates are consumed, and the food is digested and ultimately absorbed by the liver, then stored in the liver in a form called Glycogen, by a process called glycogenesis.

If there is enough glycogen in the liver, the rest is converted into fat cells. First, these fat cells are deposited in visceral areas such as the omentum, the intestine and the liver.

Insulin causes sugars to enter the body's cells, except within the brain and liver and skeletal muscles. Higher levels of insulin increase the production of fat cells.

So, the bottom line is that High insulin = More fat cells

Low insulin levels are caused by low carbohydrates and starvation.

## Starvation response

What happens with starvation?

In the initial 24 hours, glycogen is mobilized and broken down from the liver.

After 24-36 hours fat cells are broken down for energy. In addition, fats are broken down to Fatty acids and glycerol. Fatty acids are used for ketones. Major ketones are Beta Hydroxybutaric acid and acetoacetic acid. They can be used for energy by the brain and other tissues.

After 5 days of starvation ketosis sets in, protein is broken down and converted to glucose by gluconeogenesis.

## Fasting

When I tried to lose weight, it was our fasting month. I was worried as I had to fast and keep on my diet as well. I talked with friends about this, it would be so hard for me not to eat and do my fasting, but I found it was very easy, and I could do both. In fact, since I wasn't eating fried food and carbohydrates at the end of my fasting time I could do exercise and easily keep to my diet. Intermittent fasting is good way to lose weight, and I would recommend it. It can be a real help in resetting our metabolism, and getting into the habit of eating less is the key. Fasting is actually a primary factor in health, known to increase your lifespan, so in moderation is very good for you. Avoid excessive fasting though, as this can be very harmful.

## Food industry

Let us discuss the role of the food Industry.
It is one of biggest industries operating today, and has only now started to work slowly towards a healthy program. For them, it is not going to be profitable if people eat less or healthier.

For the food industry, money is the important part, not health. You can see that clearly by looking at just what we find in our food today.

## Additives

This includes substances like Fructose syrup, stemming from the commercialization of products and the introduction of fast food. I would like to point out that the food industry is a real problem, with many cases of mislabeling ingredients and the number of calories in a given food product, making it difficult for consumers to make informed choices.

# Fast food

It remains much cheaper than healthy foods, which are nearly always the most expensive choice available. Look at any sales or offers in the shopping aisles, or at a fast food chain. <u>They never have 2 salads for the price of one, they would rather give you a pie for free.</u>

## Supersize bad choices

Fast food chains will supersize drinks and meals, but never the salad.

## Serving Sizes

It's very important to pay attention to the servings sizes as well as protein carbohydrates and fat composition.

Remember to differentiate between Portion and serving size. **Serving size** is what calorie content is based off. **Portion size** is what you should eat. Most people tend to underestimate portion size. Guessing does not help. Please use weighing Scale.

## Juices Bad choices

We see lot of commercials for juices, but nothing is natural except the fruit itself.    Juice tends to remove all the goodness of real fruit, by the time juice gets to you all the good nutrients are gone; e.g. an apple, if you drink apple juice it causes your sugar levels to shoot up, but eating raw apple is healthy.

When we drink juices, we give the body an unnatural number of calories. Instead, we want to make the body work to get calories from food, if you give it raw fruit it has to work extra to digest, but if you give processed it is easier to digest and requires no work from the body.

# Principals of Diet

The basic principles of diet are simple, Intake, Output and Net Calories.

Food is composed of carbohydrates, Proteins, Fats and water. Composition of food intake is important, I mean percentage of each food type needs balance, but also the number of calories ingested matters. So, what we need to do is work out the total number of calories needed, then allocate a portion of protein and carbohydrate to our intake. This should be around 30%, but between 20% to 40% works depending on the individual, the rest of the diet should be veggies, especially greens.

Just remember to lose one pound you have to burn 3500 calories. You could divide that over the days that you would like, for example if we want to lose it over 7 days then plan to shave off 500 calories from your diet or burn 500 calories extra each day. It is just simple mathematics.

If someone tells you their metabolism is slow or fast, and they can eat as much or as little as they choose without affecting their weight, then I say to them you need to still pay attention to the mathematics of the issue.

Pay attention to the amount, serving size, portion control and the time you eat, as it all makes a difference.

Portion control is important as we stretch our stomach we cause it to get bigger and if we eat less it shrinks. The stomach has smooth muscles, and one way of causing it to enlarge is stretching.

Remember the <u>One Third rule</u>, drink one third water, eat one third food and leave one third empty.

Remember not to exceed BMR. For weight loss net should be negative.

**Stomach enlargement,** if we eat more our stomach enlarges as it gets stretched, which stimulates muscles and maintains that larger size. Do not fill up your stomach with food. Larger size of stomach difficult to maintain weight loss, I believe hormone Ghrelin levels to blame.

## Diet options

There are several diets available on the market, like no carbohydrates or high-fat high-protein diets, and some supplements for appetite suppressants to stop you feeling hungry. Remember, it is easy to lose and then gain back weight this way, this is not a short-term solution.

Most of my patients ask me about suppressing the appetite so let's work on it.

Let us overview diets. I believe the following factors contribute to failures:

**Expense:** Many diets are available today, they talk about quick fixes or tell you to buy certain products. They are always expensive.

**Short Lived:** Even if you buy the expensive products, you may lose weight in the short-term, but unfortunately gain it back again over time. You will lose water through these methods which can cause other problems and makes it an unsustainable approach.

**Appetite Suppressants**
Most of the medications used, including stimulants like Phentermine, can have cardiovascular side effects.

**Supplements** can be expensive and clinically ineffective. Check the aisles in the diet sections at stores, you will see they are expensive and full of calories.

## Ketogenic diets

the next thing to look at is the ketogenic diet. So, what is a ketogenic diet? This is a diet where you are going to eat less carbohydrates, and is based around the fact that the body will break down those stored fats into energy and free fatty acids from your body into energy in the brain tissue.

We can suppress appetite by promoting ketosis which inhibits your ability to eat so much. You can achieve that by eating less carbohydrates which we defined as less than 40 percent or between 20-40 percent a day. You can check also by using commercially available kits.

## Surgery or Quick Fix

Surgeries could help anyone lose weight quickly, generally 10-90 lbs. There are a few options such as a Lap Band, Partial or complete stomach removal. It is very effective in taking care of Type 2 diabetes, sleep apnea, arthritis and hypertension. However, there are possible complications during and after surgery, it could be a lifelong route to take and cannot be reversed so the question is, should surgery be your first choice?

I do not think so, such a permanent move should be the last resort, not the first option, in fact I have met several patients who had surgery years ago and have since put on weight again. The brain is a complicated organ, and sometimes, surgery doesn't really fix things, and over time the brain takes us back to the problem. This is why there are plenty of things to try before surgery.

## Mindful eating

This is one of the newer concepts, suggesting we need more time to eat and appreciate food. Unfortunately, many of us have developed bad habits when it comes to quick eating. We need to smell and taste food more thoroughly, as it enhances satiety and satisfaction. Even just a small amount of food is enough. I remember my teacher Jim used to ask me why I ate so fast. He told me to appreciate meta and flavors, and that was when I was overweight.

Stomach cannot differentiate between foods so if we eat our favorite food at the end stomach will still feel same and will not gain weight.

Hunger goes away if we drink some water and wait. We will eat less.

If we eat less dense foods we gain less calories, worse examples are bagels. Over the last few years food industry is trying to come up with highest calories per gram.

**Destiny**
We all are destined to eat so much in our lifetime, it is up to us if we eat in shorter time and get sick or over longer time and enjoy our life disease free.

## Poison Vs Medicine

The difference between poison and medicine is concentration. By the same principle the difference between simply eating food and becoming obese is the amount. So, if you are going to eat a lot of food then the sugars are going to make you sick, you will begin gaining a lot of weight and that's where the problems begin. Unless try to cut down the portions as well as the complexity of your food, any extra calories will start depositing gradually all over the body especially the soft tissues, such as the liver and intestines. That's the most dangerous facts, that one of the cause of belly size getting bigger is overeating, and people ask me what is the best exercise to lose that belly weight. The answer is always diet and especially limiting carbohydrates. Remember, a thin layer of fat can cover miles of intestine, so it's not going to go down quickly.

## Glycemic Index

Another concept is the glycemic index. This is the idea that a low amount of blood sugar goes up with absorption of any food, and there are a few values which I would like to discuss. The glycemic index difference between white bread and wheat bread, really is the difference of insulin secretion. It's easy for the body to handle those sugars, and then the next concept is about complex carbohydrates or simple carbohydrates. Simple carbohydrates get absorbed faster and release insulin more quickly.

Insulin promotes decreased blood sugar levels. it is good for the body because it promotes blood sugar entering into other cells all over the body, with the exception of liver brain and muscle. Insulin is also the substance that promotes low sugar fat deposits and hunger. So, we stimulate more, we will easily burn any amount of food, especially carbohydrates which makes the levels increase, and it can burn your pancreas overtime if the sugars rise too high too quickly.

## Excess Protein

Another big misconception is that if we are going to eat more protein we will be safe. The answer to that is no, and unfortunately any excess protein is also converted into whatever the body wants, including fat. It is important to remember that these basic principles never change, and through exercise or diet, and preferably both, you lose weight by having a net loss in calorie intake.

*Each night when I go to sleep, I die. And the next morning, when I wake up, I am reborn.*
*Mahatama Gandhi*

# Sleep

Let us recap about sleep.

There are two main types of sleep, Rapid Eye Movement (REM) and Non-Rapid Eye Movement (NREM), which is further divided in to Stage1, Stage 2 and Stage 3. 2/3 of our sleep is NREM and 1/3 is REM.

The best sleep is Stage 3 not REM.

The heart, brain and other organs rest during sleep, as the heart beats slower and brain neurons fire less.

REM sleep is where complications can happen.

## Sleep Apnea

Prevalence is 24 percent in men and 9percent in women by criteria of Apnea/hypopnea index above 5.

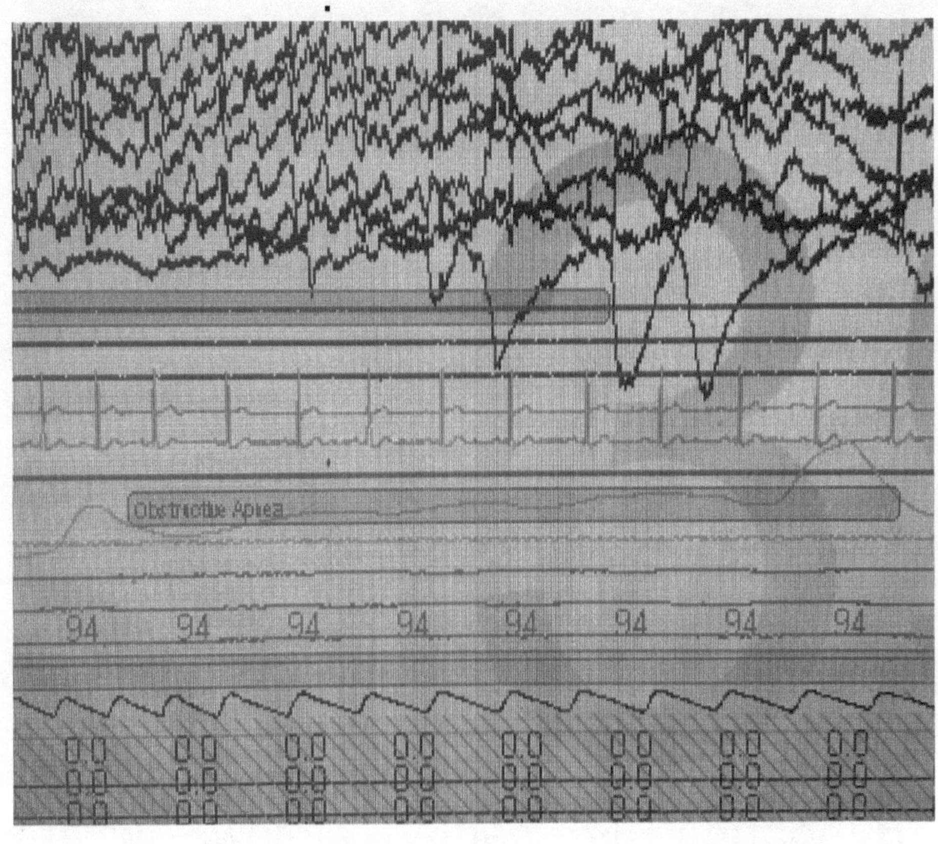



**Apnea** is when there is no airflow due to an obstruction in the upper airway, mostly behind the tongue/tonsils area, and central if no stimulation from the sleep center.

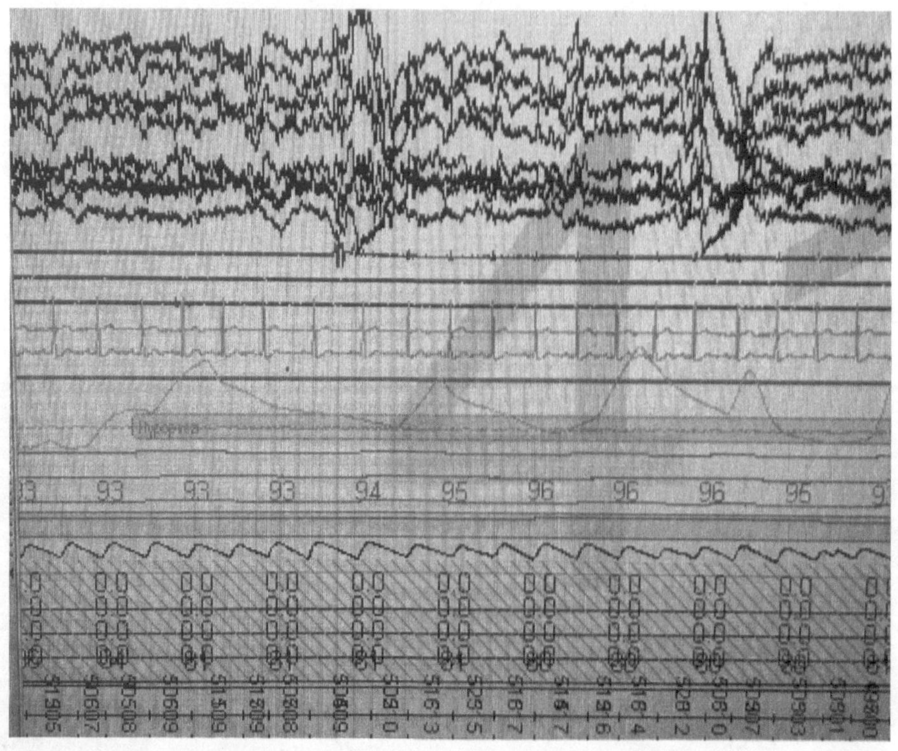

**Hypopnea** is partial airflow, where restricted flow means oxygen levels can fall a little.

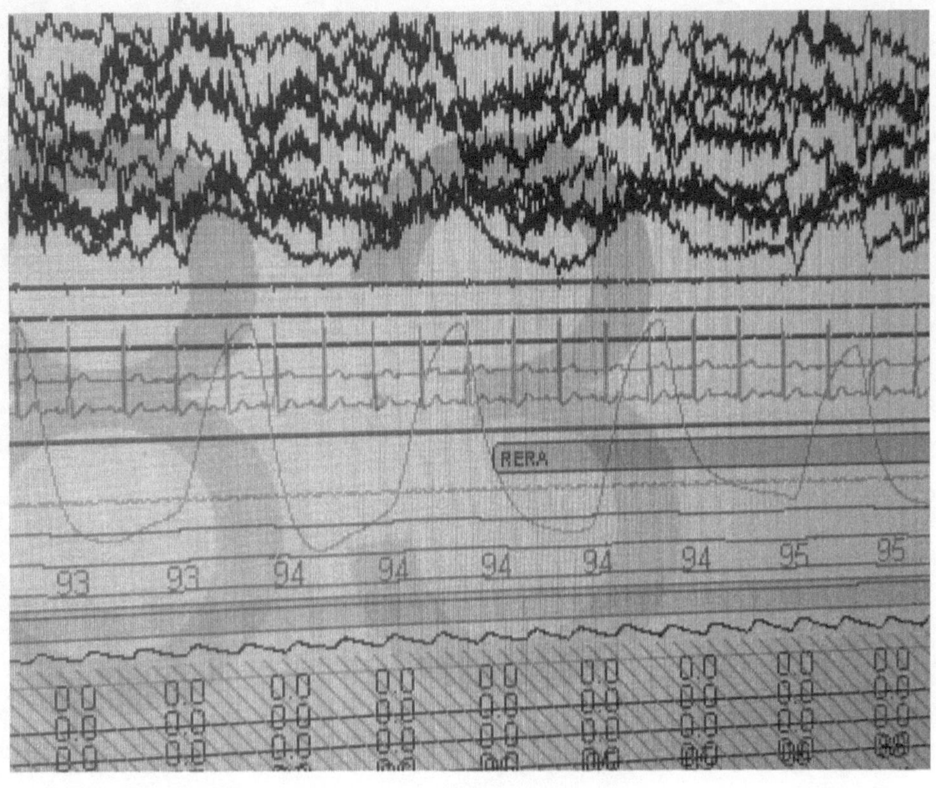


**Respiratory Effort Related Arousal (RERA)** is similar to loud snoring, and may cause brain arousals from sleep.

Arousals, which awaken the brain from sleep, can be respiratory or non-respiratory arousals. Respiratory can be from apnea, hypopnea and RERA.

Non-respiratory arousals can happen due to Leg movements, Insomnia, Acid reflux etc.

The brain has a sleep center in the hypothalamus and a wake center, or more likely network of structures in the brainstem, hypothalamus and basal forebrain.

The sleep center promotes sleep by inhibiting signals travelling to wake centers.

The same hormones, including dopamine, histamine and acetylcholine, are involved in both sleep and the Reward Center.

No wonder a lack of dopamine is associated with stress and craving for Carbohydrates.

A ten percent increase in Obesity can cause a six-fold risk of OSA.

The best time to walk is in the evening or nighttime, if you are going to do some exercise. I believe walking is pretty good exercise, especially towards the evening if you are a person who suffers from insomnia.

There is more data suggesting our sleep is affected by what we eat especially gut bacteria.

Men seem to have more Apnea, hypopneas. Women tend to exhibit more Respiratory arousal related events.

I strongly believe effects of sleep apnea on someone is strongly based on genetics. Which means same degree of sleep disturbance can effect everyone differently.

## Sleep Changes with Age

When we are young we have a lot of Stage 3 sleep, but as we grow we begin to have less and less Stage 3 deep sleep. This is especially true for men; women tend to retain some Stage 3 sleep throughout life. Men lose this kind of sleep much faster. Women will wake up more often in the night than men, so in the morning women will often feel less rested even if they had a deeper sleep. Testosterone makes our sleep worse and estrogen improves it.

Connection with weight

Obesity contributes toward Obstructive sleep apnea as airways; especially the oral /pharyngeal area is narrowed. Fat deposits narrow it, and if the neck size over17 is a risk factor for this situation. Sleep apnea can cause sleepiness and fatigue, and to stimulate ourselves we crave Carbohydrates as they tend to make us feel better, but then as a result we gain weight. So, we have to break this cycle to successfully lose weight. Sleep apnea is snoring when asleep, and the throat can get narrowed or obstructed, causing brief periods that stop breathing altogether. These episodes can either mean you quit breathing completely, which is apnea, or there is hypoxemia (which means Low Oxygen) where you partially quit breathing.

This is one of the most feared complications with sleep, and when you have low oxygen it puts your heart at fight mode and it causes an adrenaline rush while sleeping. So, it is detrimental for the heart, as it increases oxygen consumption, making the heart work all night instead of resting, and this especially problematic when switching from NREM to REM state. The release of a lot of adrenaline causes many problems for the heart, such as arrhythmias and even cardiac death can happen. This is crucial, and we must realize the connection. There is strong association with high blood pressure, enlarged heart or cardiomyopathy to name just a few.

Sleep apnea and weight gain. I have a lot of patients who have gained weight and felt tired and have severe carb cravings due to sleep apnea. We must realize that with sleep apnea we will be craving for carbohydrates more as they are stimulating, making you active for a short time. But they also make weight issues worse, so we gain more weight and the sleep apnea gets worse. The solution is to get treated, and then enjoy more energy and lose weight quickly.

Sleep apnea is an important cause of heart arrhythmia. In my case, may be cause of my PVC's (premature Ventricular Contractions) or extra beats. Over the years, I have observed important cause of recurrent atrial fibrillation or an irregular heartbeat.

Shift workers can quickly gain weight, as it is known fact that workers working at night tend to eat more. If you are night time worker pay attention to your calories.

Sleep eating disorder is another one where people will get up and eat and then go to bed. We have to keep this in mind if we have unexplained disorder.

Other disorders include Narcolepsy (excessive sleepiness), Kluver- Bucy Syndrome.

In my opinion all weight loss programs really benefit from sleep apnea treatment.

By the same token if with weight loss, the sleep apnea also goes away. It is cured.

Insomnia is inability to fall or remain asleep. Inadequate sleep hours and or quality lead to fatigue and possible weight issues. It can be acute due to any event or chronic when it lasts over 6 months.

Insomnia is mostly caused by behavioral issues and chronic pain. We need to address those before things can improve.

Insomnia can cause increased Grehlin and lower Leptin as you recall

<u>Grehlin can increase appetite and Leptin can lower it.</u>

People with insomnia can have hyperarousal state. They usually do not nap. As you recall, brain has different parts, they work best when work in rhythm. If someone has hyperarousal state it puts lot of stress on brain. I strongly believe relaxation techniques help.

Insufficient sleep is most common especially in teenagers. I recommend that all my patients get enough and better-quality sleep. There are a few things can affect sleep, and we will go over each so you can see clearly where the problems may be.

Remember try to get 6-8 hours of sleep. For teenagers and younger patients more sleep is recommended over 9 hours.

Try to change your habit by dedicating time for your thoughts for example late afternoon one hour instead in the bed.

Acid Reflux

Sleep and reflux can cause real problems together. We have a tendency to eat and then to sleep, and so we often like to eat heavily just so we can fall asleep. This is one of the worst things we can do for number of reasons. My patients would often try to fill up their stomachs and that can cause all kinds of issues. We need to remember that's only time the body will try to rejuvenate, and digest food.

We need four hours to process our food and get our body ready for the next digestive phase. But what happens when we eat heavy, is that a full stomach can cause acid reflux, which means stomach contents including food and acid moves up the digestive tract. Stomach acid peaks between 10 PM and 2 AM and during sleep this can cause hyper acidity.

Sleep apnea can be made worse too, as food might irritate the junction of the esophagus or food pipe with the throat.

What happens is that basically your food has to be absorbed by the body, but as the stomach's digestion system slows down as we sleep, blood sugar levels can rise significantly. This can cause issues, leaving your muscles unable to work properly and making sleep apnea worse. Remember, if you have time in the evening, do some mild exercise, walking is a pretty good exercise to do that most people can easily manage. If you are a person who suffers from insomnia try to exercise in the evening, it can really help. Nature always knows best, for instance if you try to feed birds in the evening, they will never eat any food no matter what you give them, so why we should be eating heavily before we go to sleep?

**Sleep Apnea treatments** include Continuous Positive Airway Pressure or (CPAP) and Bilevel Positive Airway Pressure (BIPAP). In simple terms it is splinting of your narrow airway using room air. Other options include Oral devices. Untreated sleep apnea can cause problems with heart especially hypertension. I have seen more problems with rhythm especially extra beats or Paroxysmal Ventricular contractions PVC's and Atrial fibrillation or irregular rhythm. Other useful tips are weight management, nasal allergies control, use of wedge or incline head side of bed.

**For Insomnia,** try to maintain regular sleep schedule and do relaxation techniques most of chronic insomnia is maladaptive behavior which we have to address. Try to wake up same time, avoid late nights and keep bed only for sleep. Addressing and managing stress and mood disorders is the key. I always encourage people to maintain schedule wake up time, try to get some blue sky exposure during day which helps to reset brain.

Keep your bedroom especially your bed for sleep only. Which means no TV, phone. Do not remain in bed over 45 minutes if unable to sleep. Brain remembers every night which we are unable to sleep just like hard drive.

Avoid bright lights especially blue spectrum near bed time.

Medications are only for temporary relief. Induced sleep is never as good as our natural sleep.

I always tell people look at birds and animals they maintain such rhythm and do not need medications.

**Meditation,** couple of times a day especially evening is helpful. I postulate that few minutes of mediation actually similar to deep sleep in resetting brain. I use walking for relaxation it works and you can add meditation to it.

### Excessive sleepiness

Hypersomnia especially Narcolepsy is under reported. As a result, lot of patients think they are just lazy or slow, but I highly recommend to see Doctor. Our brain has some areas which can be referred to (sleep center) and (wake center). Awake state is more of function of areas versus one area, but still some areas are more prominent. Refer to picture. Certain neurotransmitter such as Orexin deficiency stabilizes both sleep and Awake states. Deficiency can result in Narcolepsy. More common in teenagers.

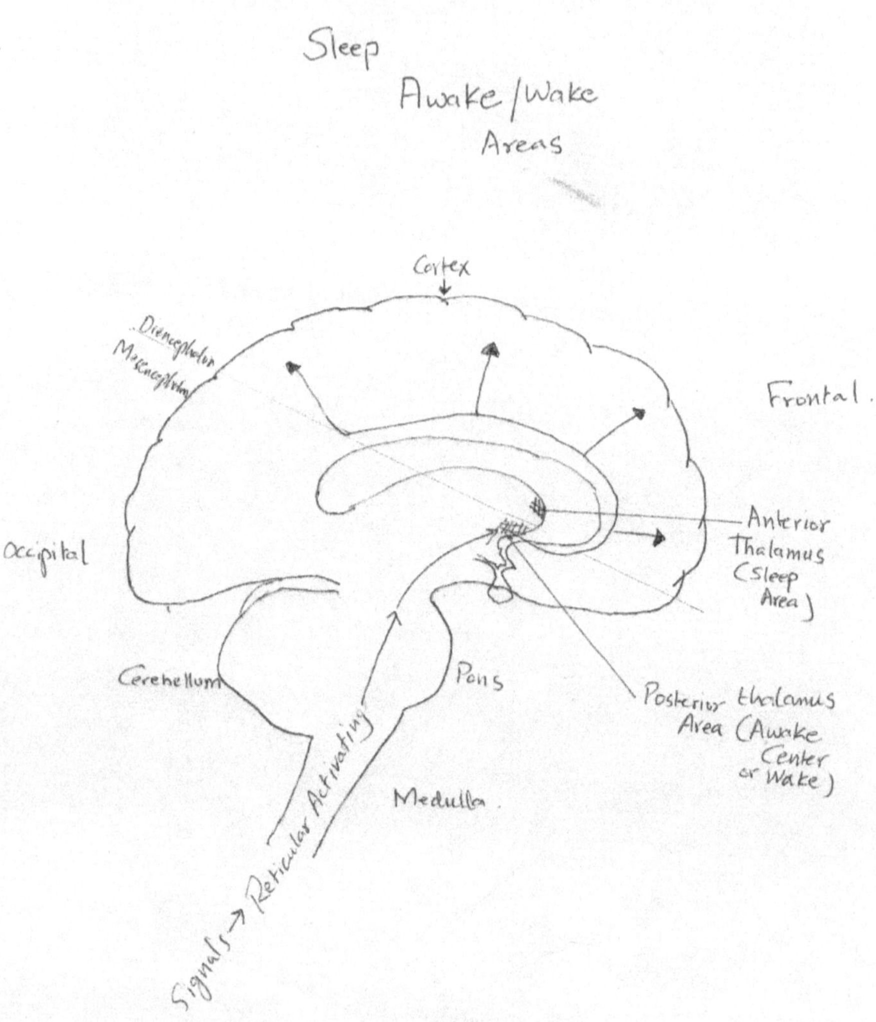


# Sleep/ Wake Areas Brain

**Circadian Rhythm**

especially Shift work disorders are also very important. Our brain has intrinsic clock which regulates irrespective of outside clock. For example, if we are in spaceship our brain clock runs approximately 24.2 hours +/- for male/female. It keeps on drifting clockwise fashion. It needs external clues to synchronize to 24 hrs. It depends on period of light especially blue wavelength and night time. Melatonin secretion helps to maintain it. Light exposure can effect melatonin and subsequent rhythm. Shift workers have higher chances of weight issues and sleep problems. Old saying still true Early to bed and early to rise make you healthy wealthy and wise.

## Failures

We are all afraid of failures, I think it helps to fine tune if you keep working on it. I think we could end up feeling disheartened because of it. If I eat more food, what I usually do to remedy things is simply to do more exercise that day.

**Cheating** can consist of going over the amount or type of food eaten. For the amount try to eat proteins or veggies in larger quantities, you can cheat once a week but try to eat food which is good.

If you eat wrong type of food, such as more carbohydrates, then try to eat complex carbohydrates. If you really have to eat bad carbohydrates then eat the smallest amount to satisfy you.

Exercise extra if you have to balance it.

# Exercise

Next thing which is very important is exercise, and there are a few things very important about exercise when it comes to weight loss.

## Consistency

So, whatever you do try to do it every day. Figure out a way to fit it into your busy schedule regularly every day, it can be difficult, I know, but it will be worth it.

## Intensity

The other thing is intensity, which is important as you really don't need to spend money on buying equipment to exercise, simply walking 30 minutes is pretty good as long as you do it consistently. The other thing is that this kind of exercise is gentle on joints and avoids long term problems. Also, you don't need to lift weights, but if you do. make sure you can maintain that weight program every day.

## Interval training

Another area to look at for exercise is interval training,      it promotes good cholesterol which is high density lipoprotein or HDL. I remember my HDL was 29 with a high carb diet, and then I was able to improve it in four days with some exercise to 60 without medication. That's why it's very important we don't ignore exercise when we look at weight loss.

It will really help those day when we cheat or eat more than our routine.

Target heart rate is the maximum achieved with exercise, calculated by the following formula: 210-age. If you achieve 60% of max target it is cardio exercise, if you keep 40-60 % it is fat burning.

When you lose weight, you become lighter and burn less calories so adjust exercise accordingly.

Machines give wrong information about calories for example you burn average of 100 calories for one mile run at 5mph with an incline.

**Strength Exercises**

Some are Dead lifts using 5-25 pounds with gradual progression.

Squats, using 5 to 25 lbs.

Pushups 3 sets of 10

Pull ups, set of 10

Core Strengthen by

Planks possibly the best

Scissors

Leg lifts

**Yoga,** best for people with joint issues.

**I found simple easy walking few miles before going to bed is more**

**<u>relaxing and effective than running. Add some meditation to it.</u>**

## <u>Advantages  of walking</u>

1. No equipment needed. Can do indoor/outdoor.
2. Easy to do any time
3. More relaxing especially evening.
4. Gentle on body.
5. Can still listen to music, meditate and even work
6. Count steps manually e.g. 2600 steps equal 1 mile.
7. Incorporate in your daily routine.

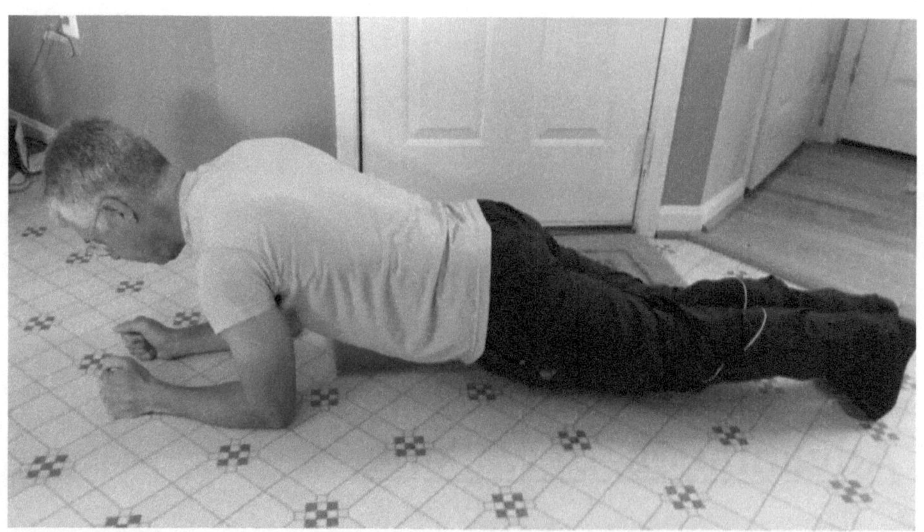

## Planks

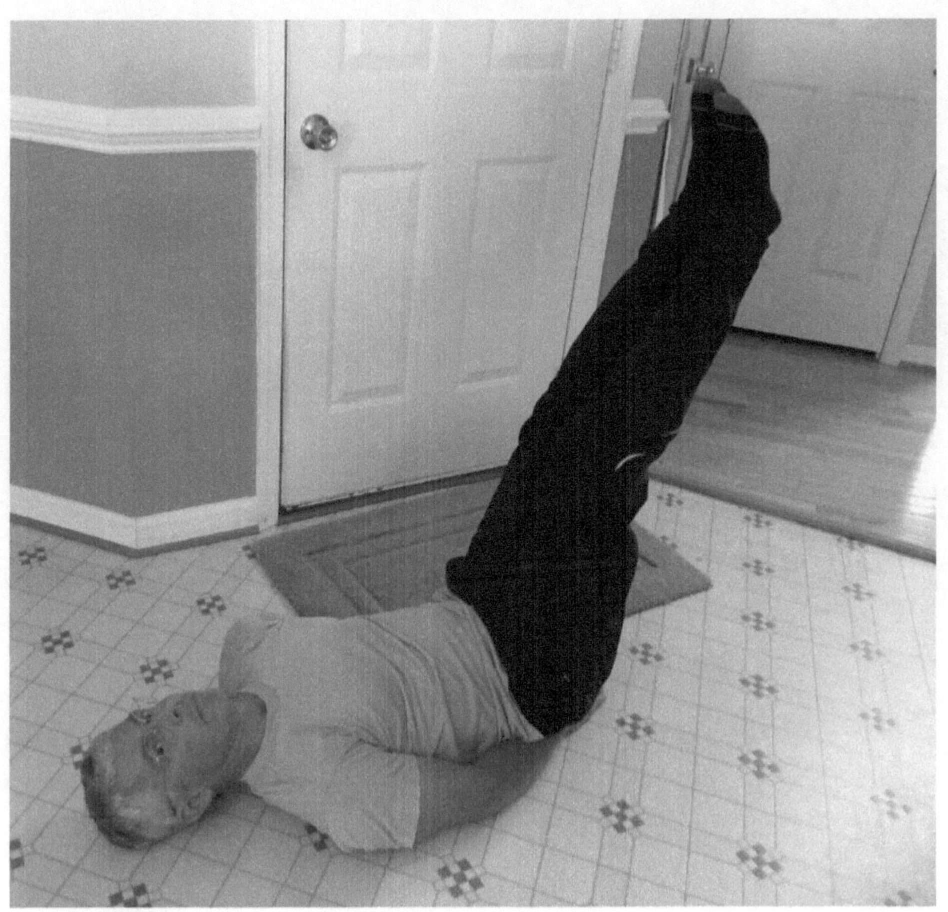

Leg lifts

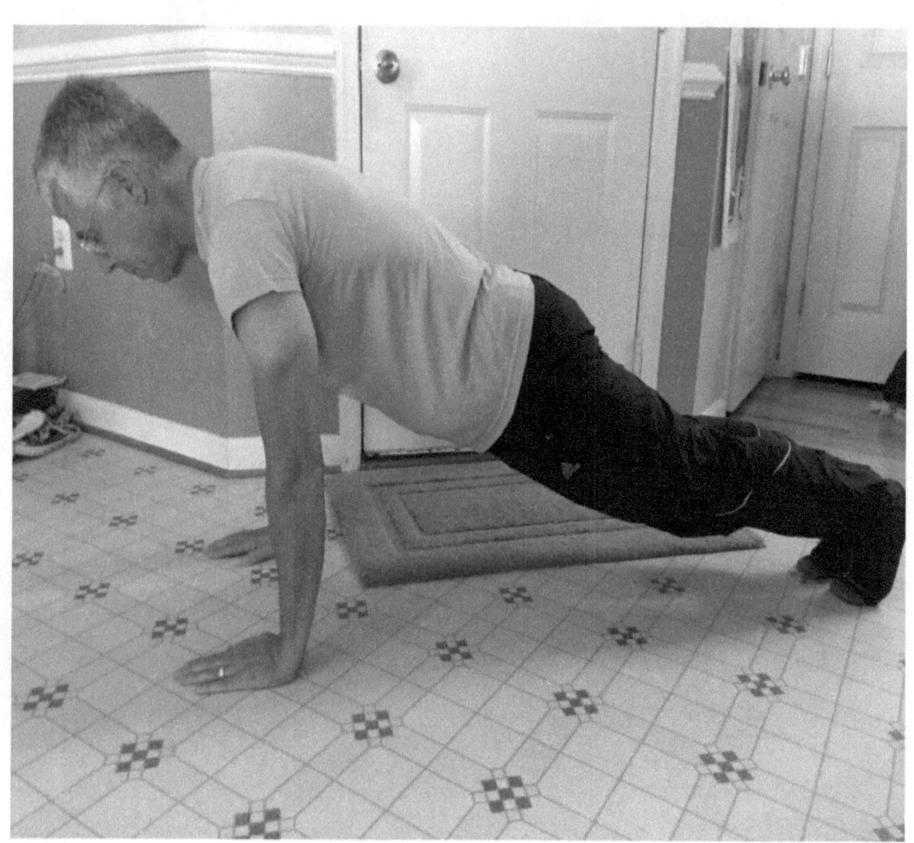

Planks

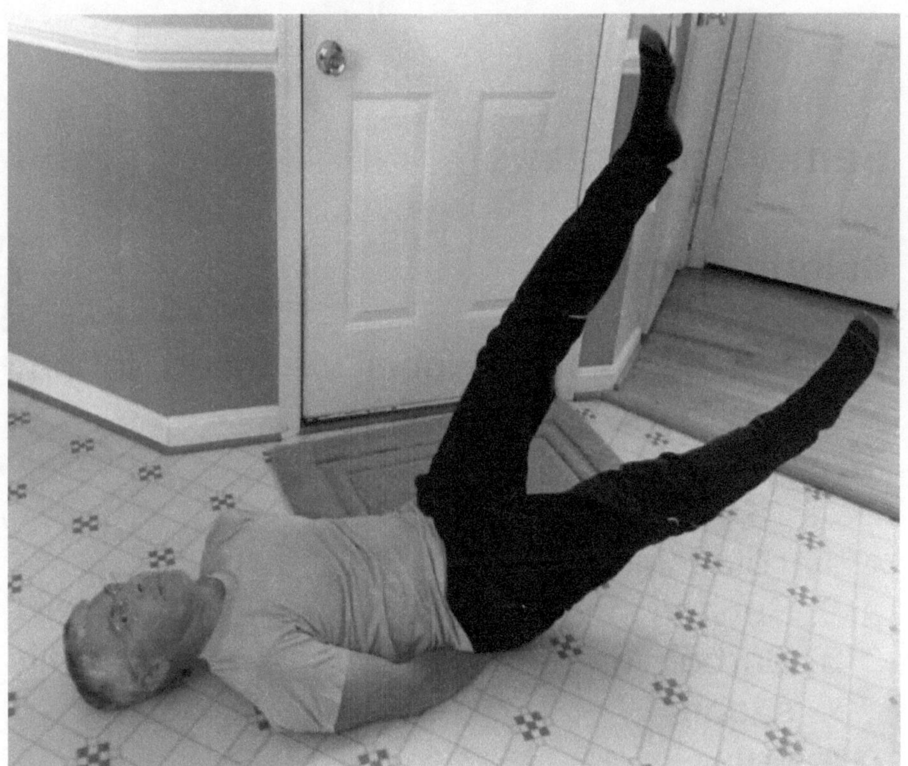

Flutter kicks

# Sample diet plans

## Calorie guide

When we look at a label we need to pay attention to the following:

1. Total calories
2. Serving size
3. Carbohydrate percentage, especially sugars
4. Fats
5. Protein

Example
See other page

# NUTRITION FACTS

Serving Size 1 Cup (240mL)
Servings Per Container 8

**Amount Per Serving**

| | |
|---|---|
| **Calories** 90 | Calories from Fat 0 |

**% Daily Value***

| | |
|---|---|
| **Total Fat** 0g | **0%** |
| Saturated Fat 0g | **0%** |
| *Trans* Fat 0g | |
| **Cholesterol** <5mg | **1%** |
| **Sodium** 125mg | **5%** |
| **Potassium** 410mg | **12%** |
| **Total Carbohydrate** 13g | **4%** |
| Dietary Fiber 0g | **0%** |
| Sugars 12g | |
| **Protein** 8g | **17%** |

**Recommended veggies:**

Lettuce - both iceberg and butter
Cucumbers
Mushrooms
Cilantro
Raw onion
Spinach
Lemon
Broccoli

**Dressings:**

Vinegar
Lemon

**Meats**
Fish:
Trout
Salmon limited
Flounder

Goat - lean
Lamb - lean

Beef
Turkey - limited due to salt
Smoked meats - limited due to salts
Quail
Cheese

**Limited Yogurt,**

Egg plant
Zucchini
Limited Cabbage

Avoid chickpeas, humus, mayo

Avoid Tomatoes, Rice, Bread, Crotons, corn

**Fruits:**

Apples
Oranges (but preferably use one of them)
Kiwi

Avoid grapes and mangoes

This is one of the diets on which I lost weight steadily, at a rate of 2-3 lbs. per week. I will share it with everybody

**Breakfast:**

Three egg whites with 50g chicken

**Lunch:**

 100g of chicken, turkey or shrimp with lettuce and cucumbers.

**Dinner:**

200g of chicken, barbecued fish, lamb/goat or cheese with lettuce and cucumbers

My Carbohydrates were 30 percent per day

Protein was 40 percent
Veggies was 40percent

Exercise goal 30 min daily walking


One thing I tried was chicken tandoori, which was great for me because it provided 30 g of protein each serving and was easy to eat and cook. Another thing I tried and would recommend was ground beef, which really helped to keep in shape. Grilled shrimp with some salsa was also a good dish.

Egg white is interesting. Now, you can have unlimited egg whites, but no egg yolk. If you feel hungry, eat eggs or chicken and add more lettuce and cucumber. You can have unlimited amounts of those, my choice was iceberg lettuce, but also I like butter lettuce.

<u>**Foods (I ate)**</u>

**Breakfast:** Eggs, cucumber, walnuts
**Calories 150, Carbs 3gm, Fat10gm,
Protein 14gm**

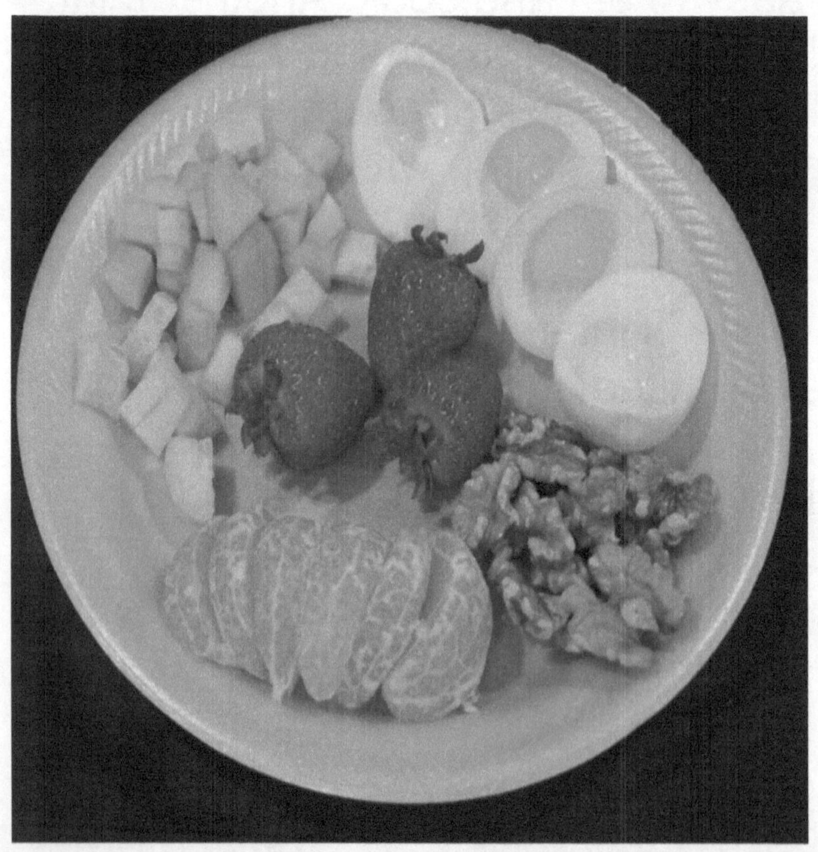

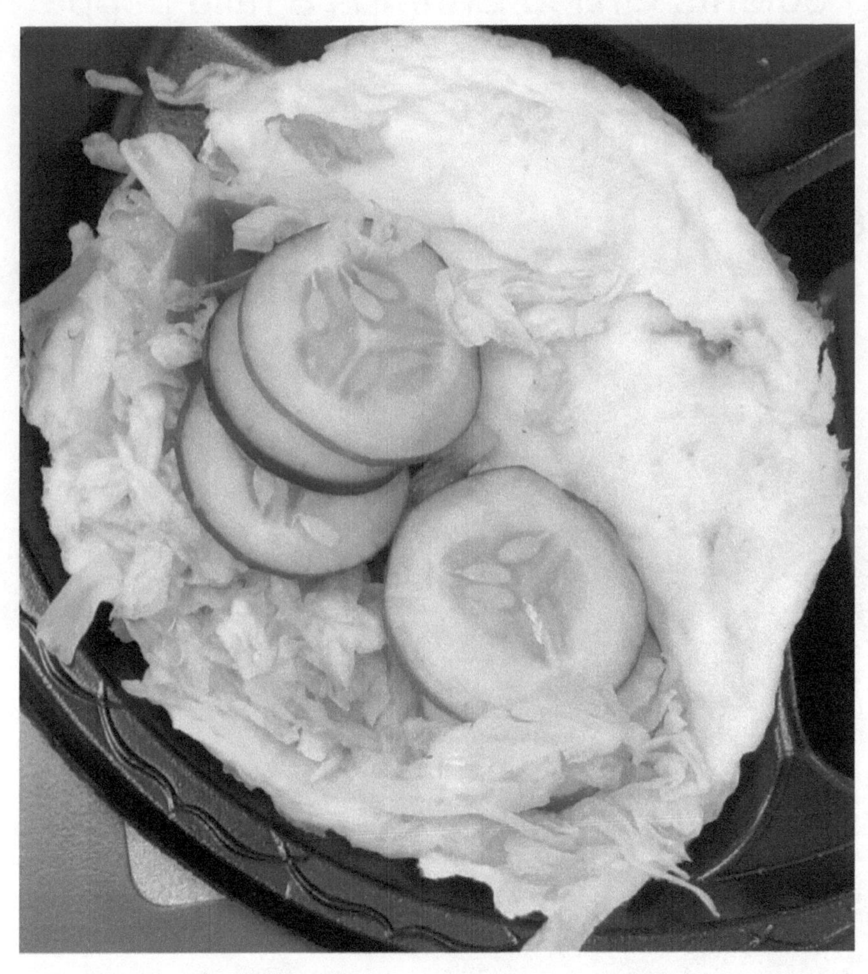

## Breakfast/Anytime Energizer

Egg white with cucumbers and lettuce

**Cal 34, Carbs 0.2g, Fats 0.1g, Protein 3.6g**

Ingredients Grilled Shrimps 8 mild pepper
seasoning
Cucumbers
Lemon
cilantro

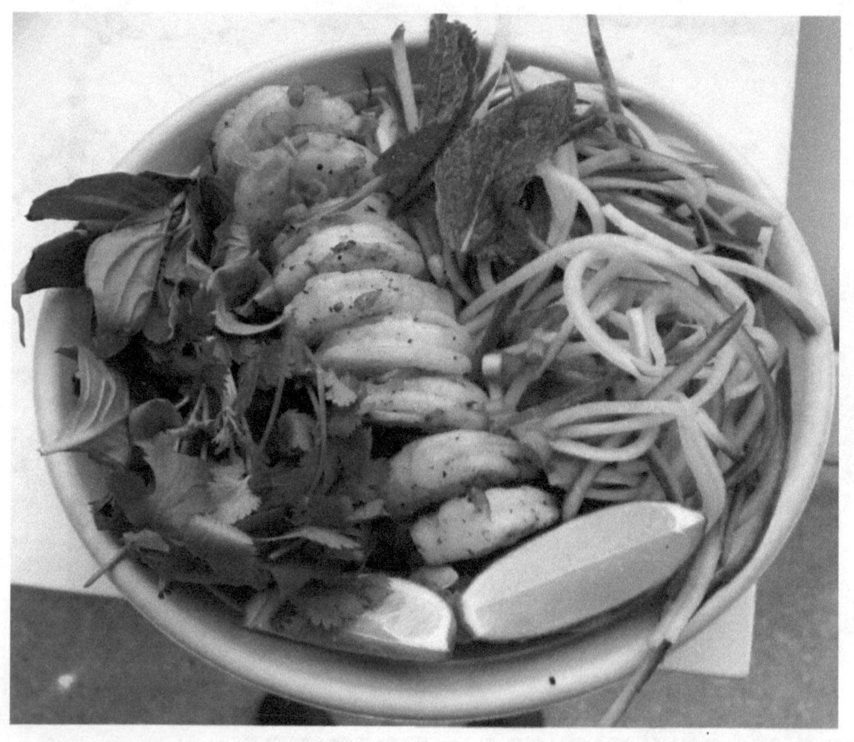

Grilled Shrimp 3.5oz, **Cal150, Fat 1.5,
Carbs 0**

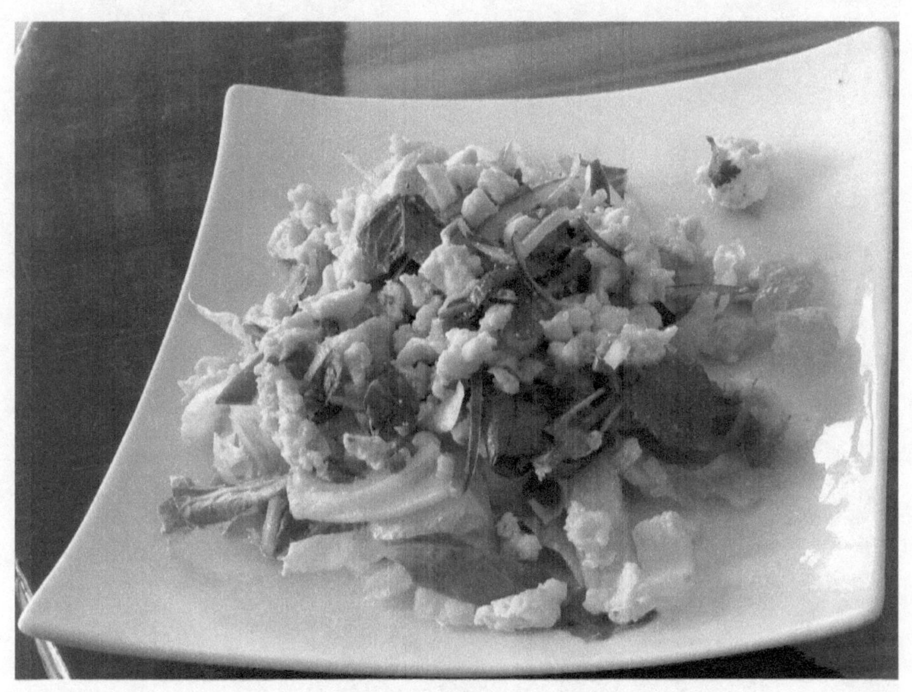

Thai chicken salad 235 minus thai sauce
**0.5 salad, Carbs 3g, fat10g, protein 8g**

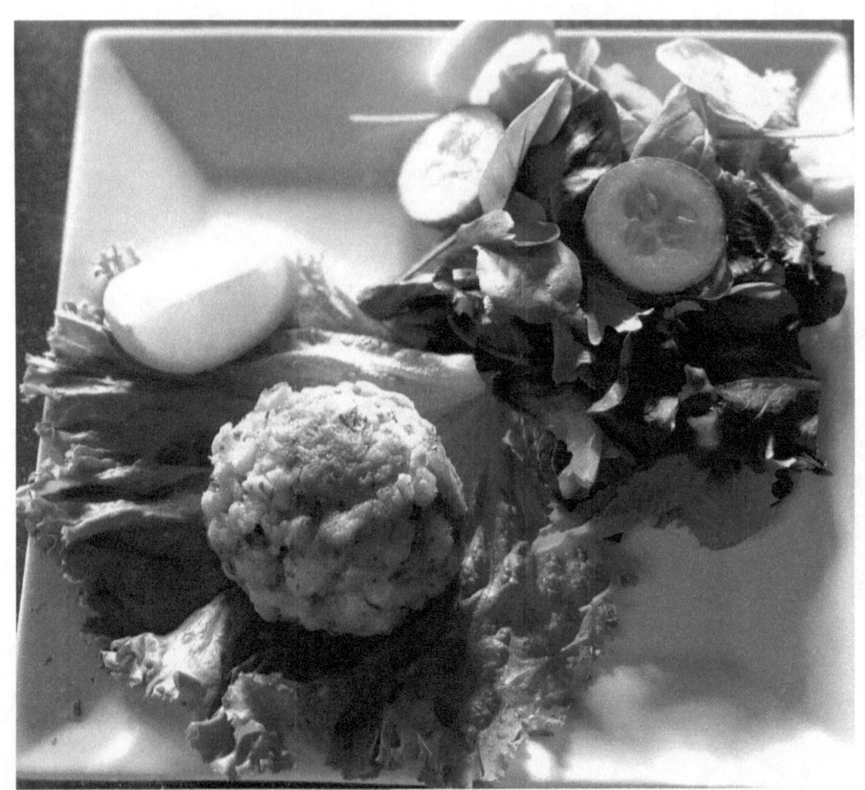

Crab Cake grilled no butter
**Cals 88/2 oz, 2.1g carbs, 6g fat, protein 6.4g**

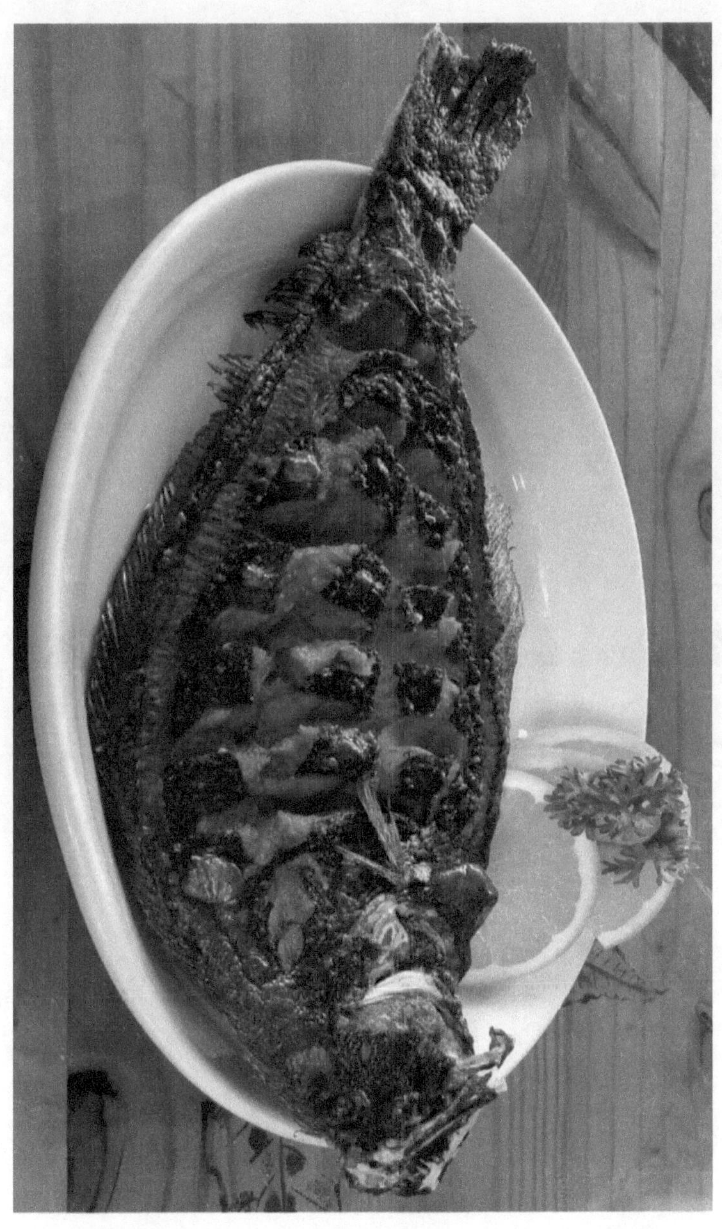

Thai fish cal 267/5 oz
**Carbs 9g, Fat 15.2 g, Pro22.4**

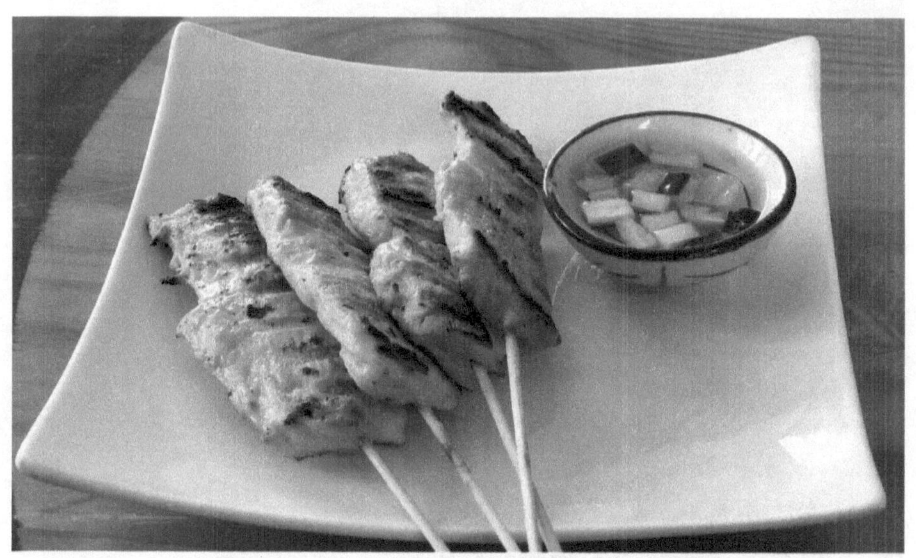

Thai Chicken 69 cals/stick No sauce
**Carbs 2.7g, Fat 6.2g, Protein 0.9g**

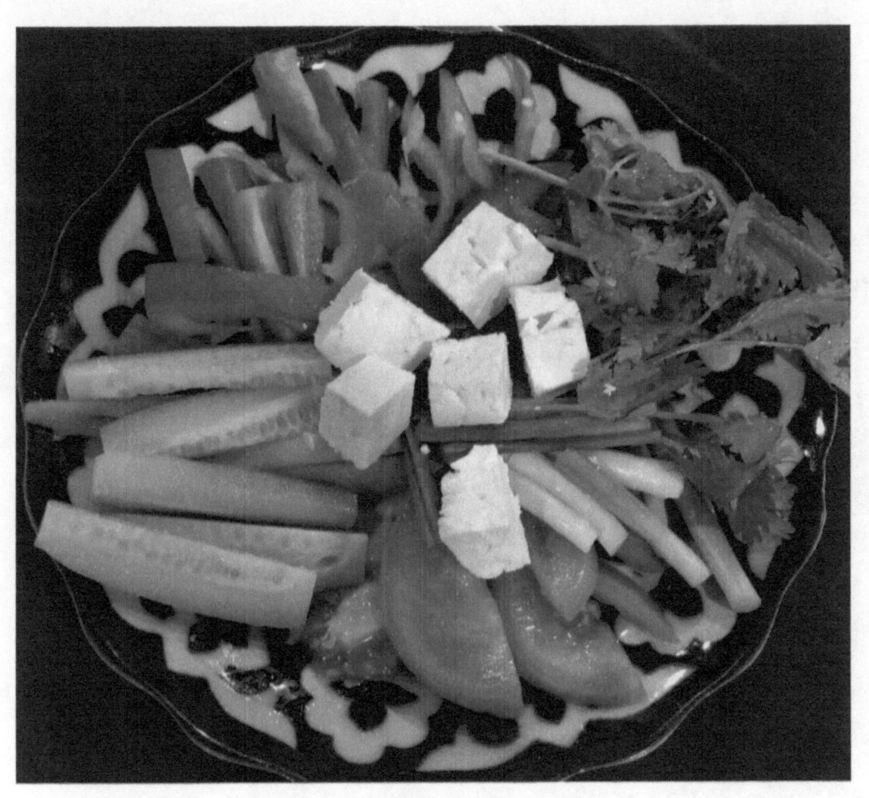

Salad  **Cal 100, Prot 7g, carb 9g, fat 4.5g**

Cucumbers, Cheese Feta1oz, cilantro, pepper100g

Ingredients
Lettuce wraps, Lettuce, Cucumbers
Cabbage leaves, Cilantro
Grilled Chicken 200gm white

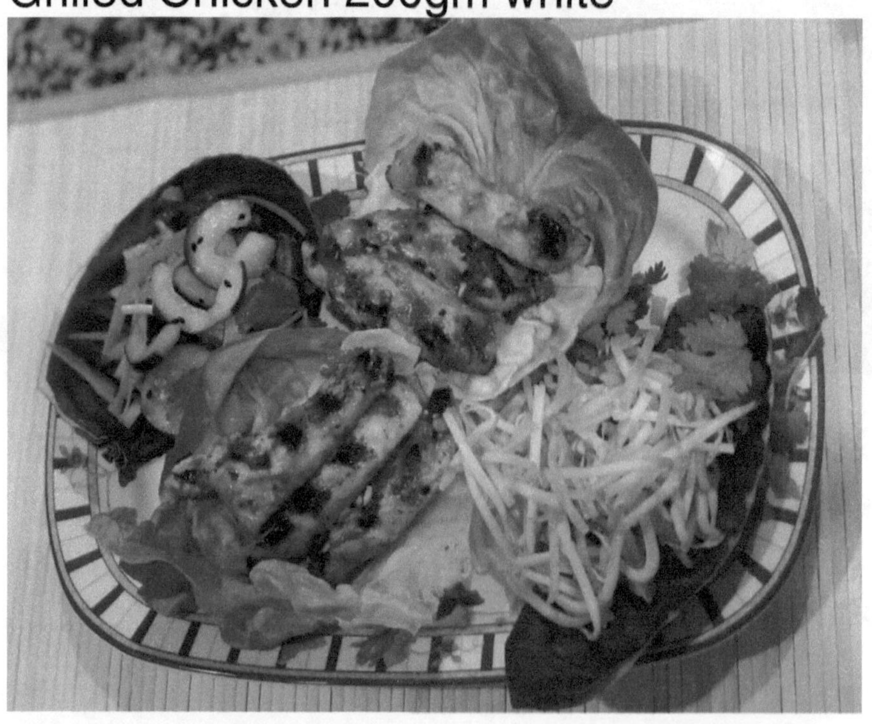

**Cal 200, Carbs 1g, Fat 4.1g, Protein 25.7**

Steak Salad 155 Cal
Steak  3  oz,  lettuce,  Bell  pepper,Salsa
**Prot 18g, Carb 2g, Fat 6g**

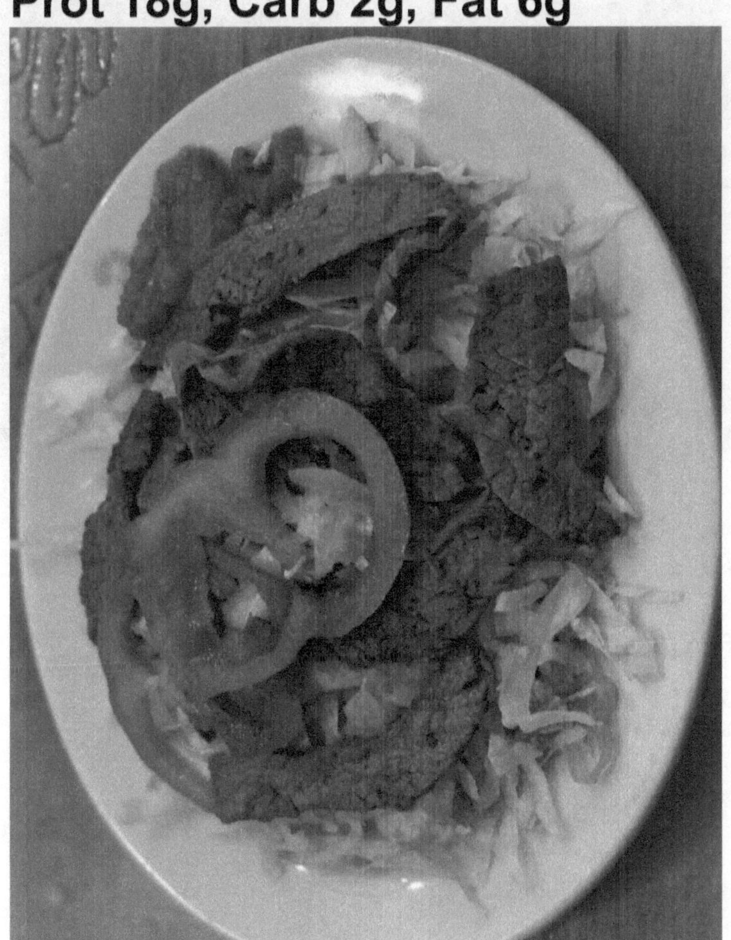

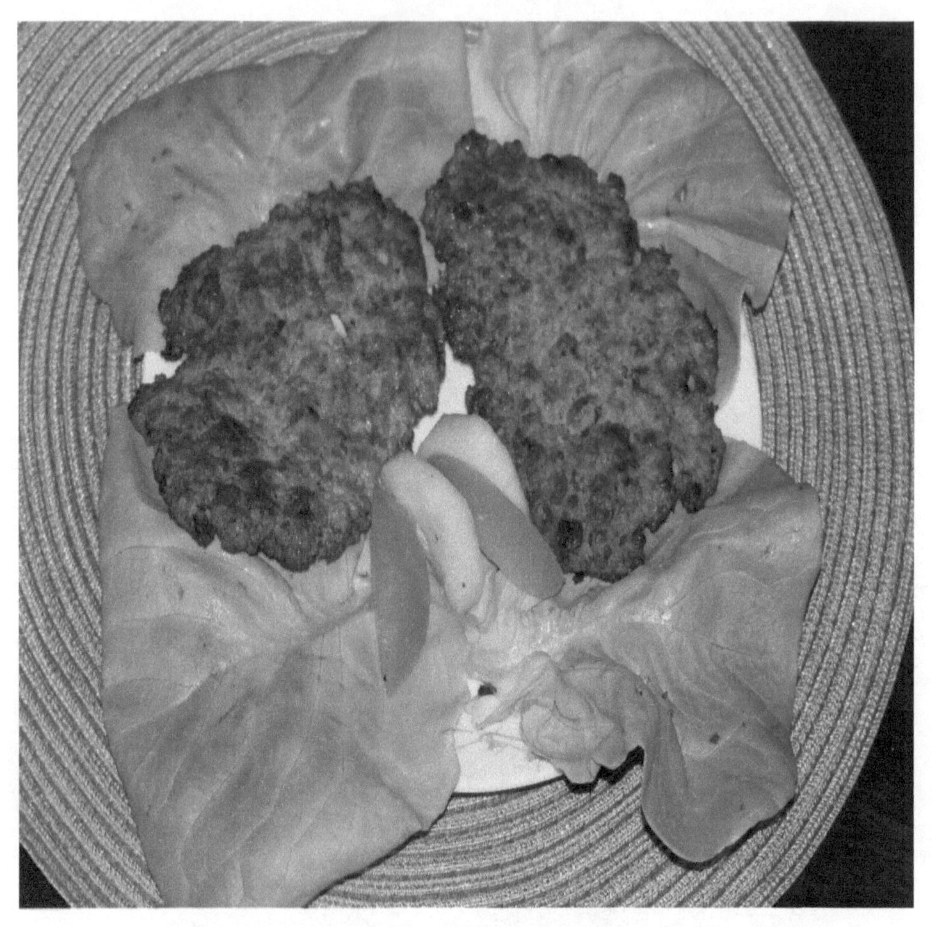

Beef Chapli Kabob **200gm Protein 9g, fat 7g, Carbs 6g, Cal 240**

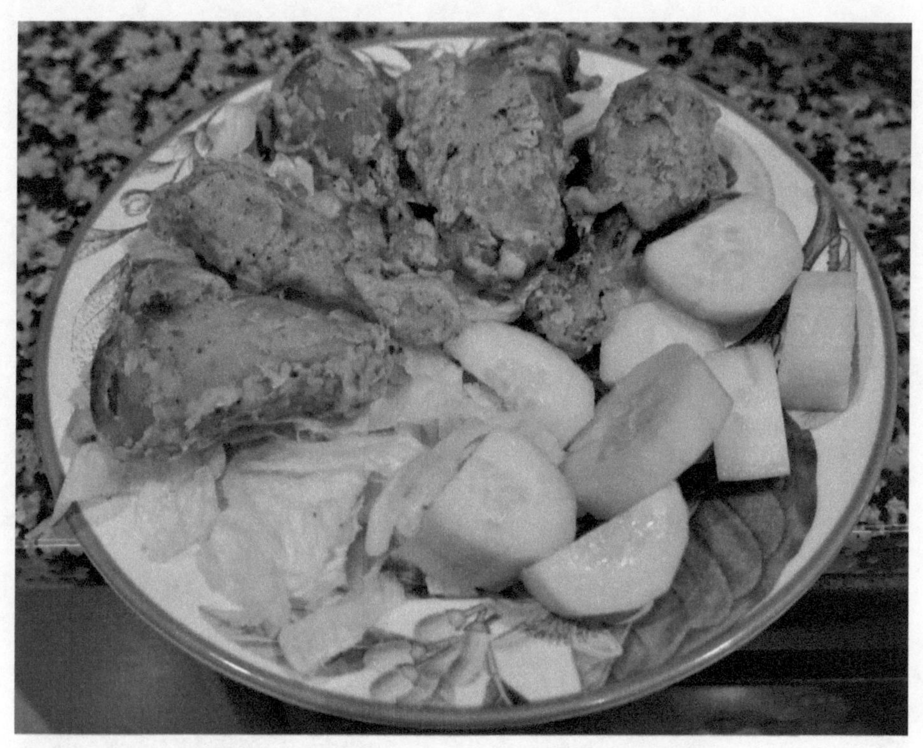

**Size 200gm, Calories 190, Carbs 2g, Fat 3.6, Protein 31g**

Chicken Broast

# Lamb Chops
**Size 3oz, Calories 250g, Carbs 0, Fat 18g, Protein 21g**

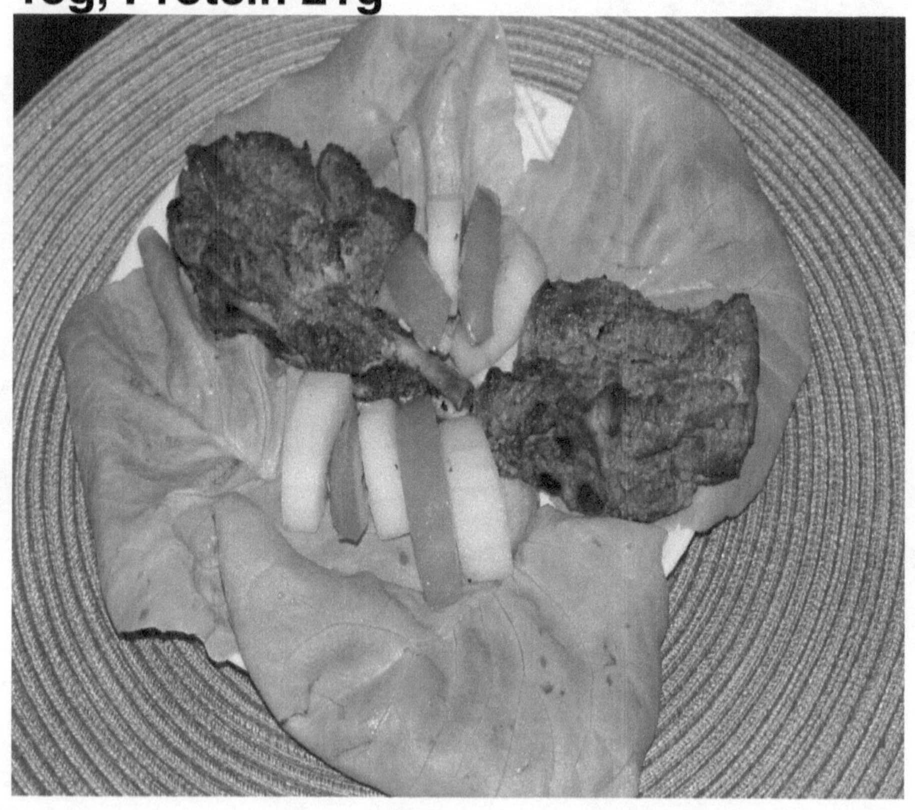

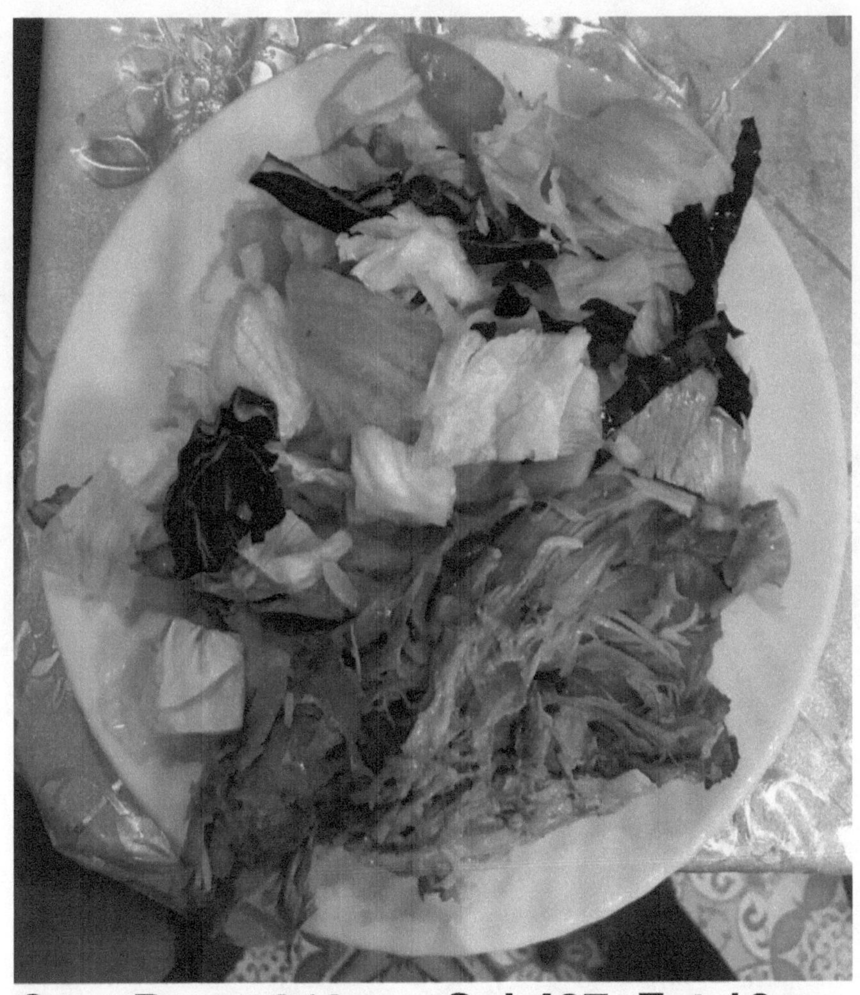

Goat Roast 340gm, **Cal 487, Fat 10gm, Protein 90gm, carbs none**

# Chicken Charcoal
## Cal 290 4oz
## 24gm protein, 22g fat, Carbs 0g

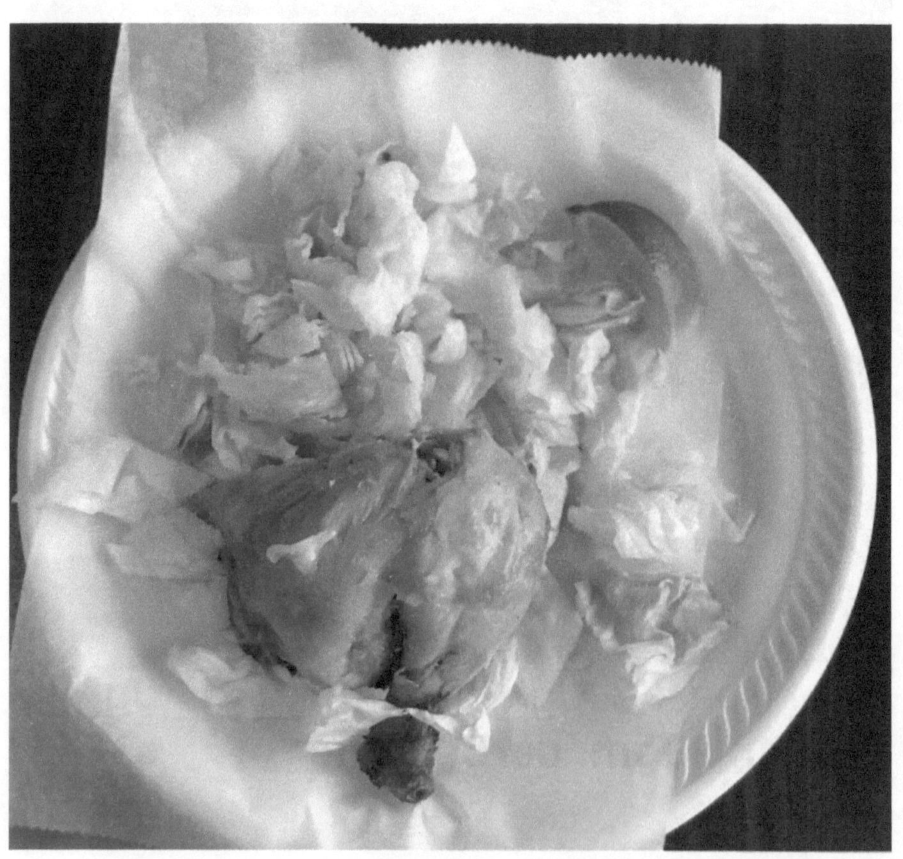

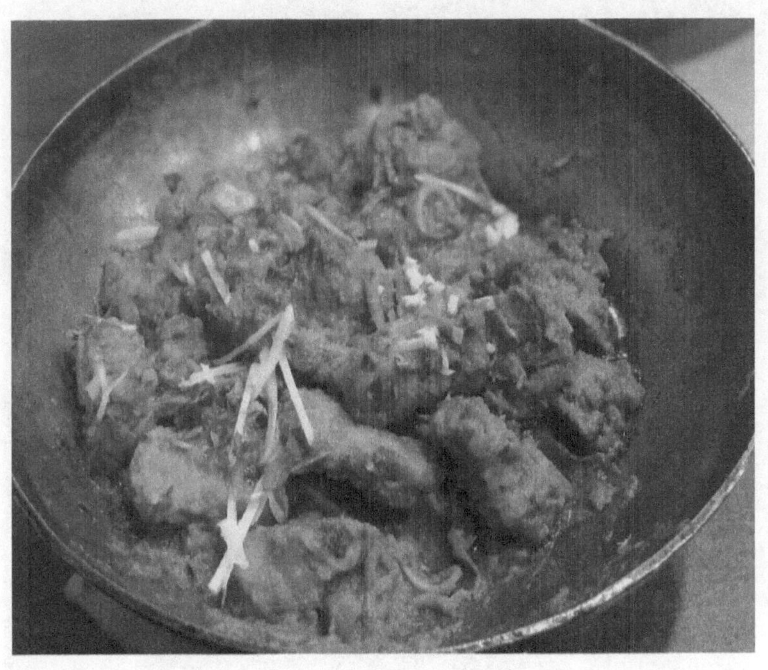

Goat karahi, 100gm boneless
**Cal 262, carbs 1.5g, fat 21.9g, Protein 18.1g**

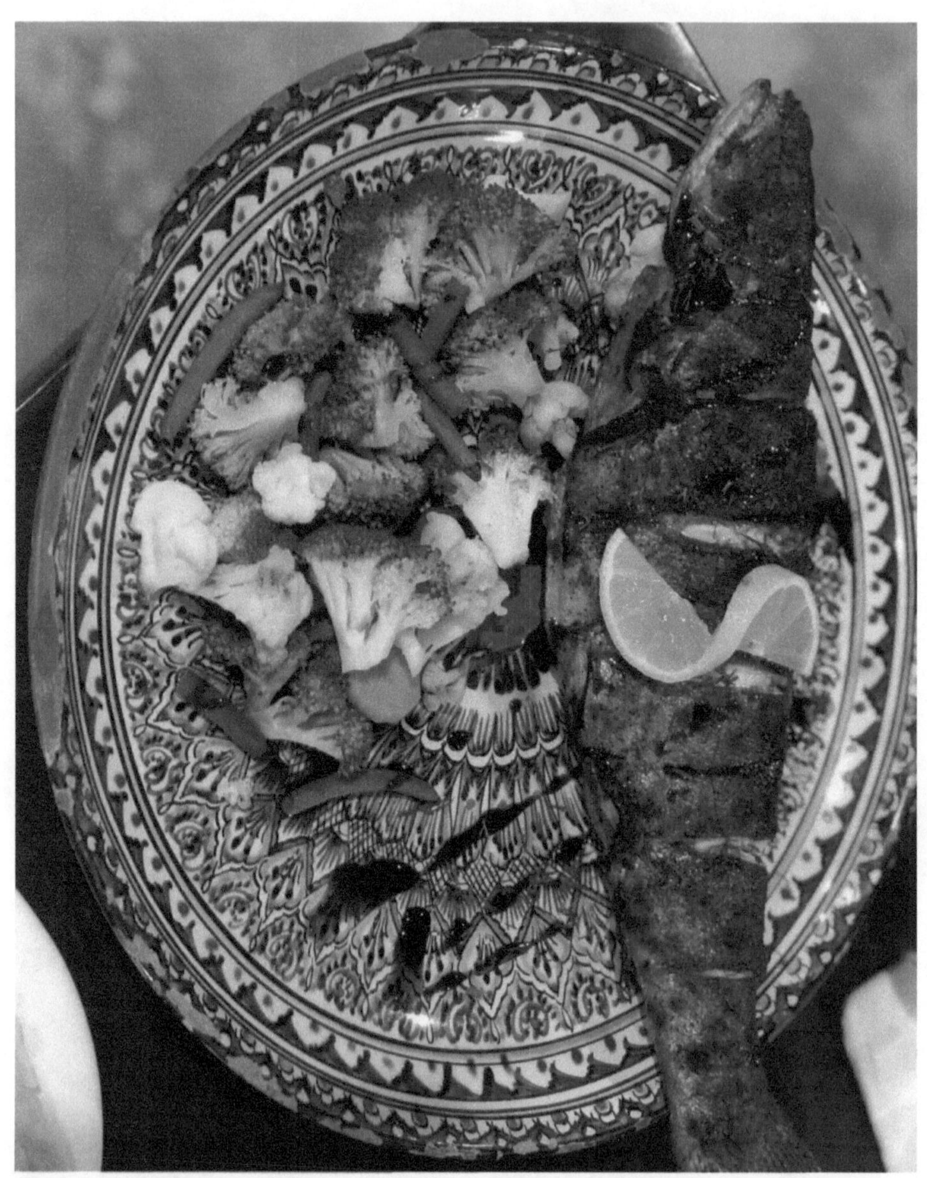

BakedTrout Cals150, 4oz w/o bones
**1g carbs, Fat 7g, Protein 21g**

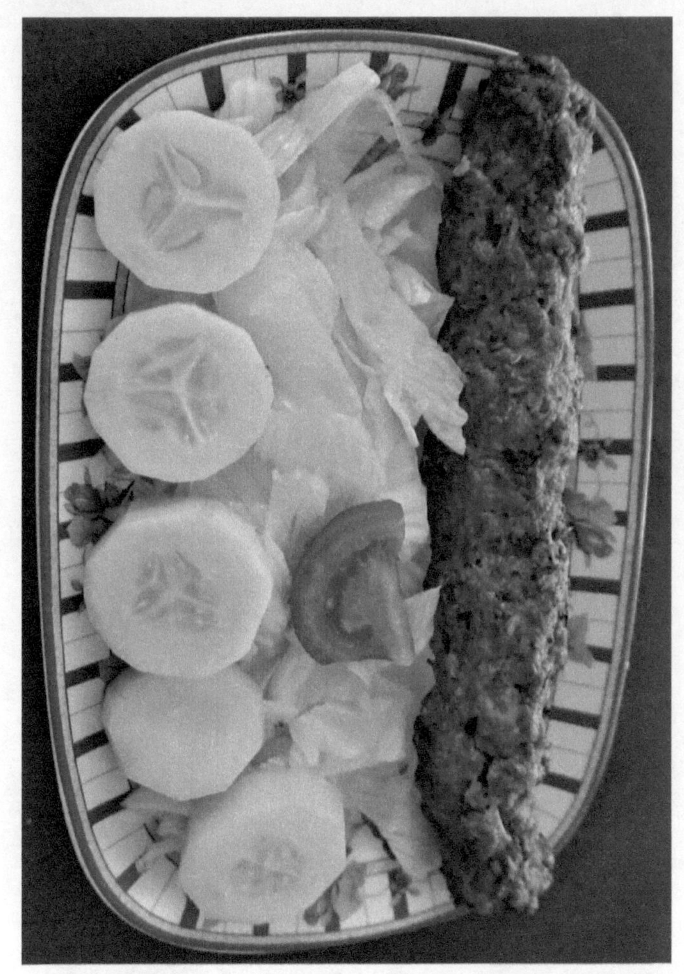

Seekhkabob**160Cals/3Oz Carbs2g,Fat10.8g, Protein13g**

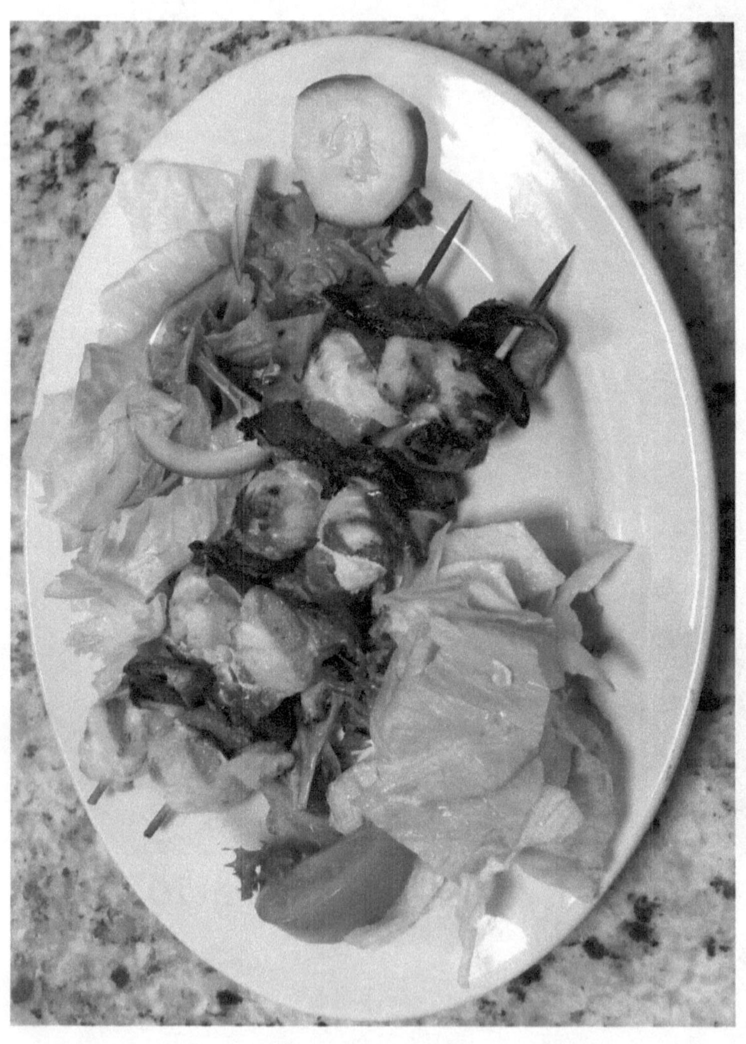

Shish Kobob Chicken per skewer/**150cals, Carbs 6g, Fat1.5g, Protein 28g**

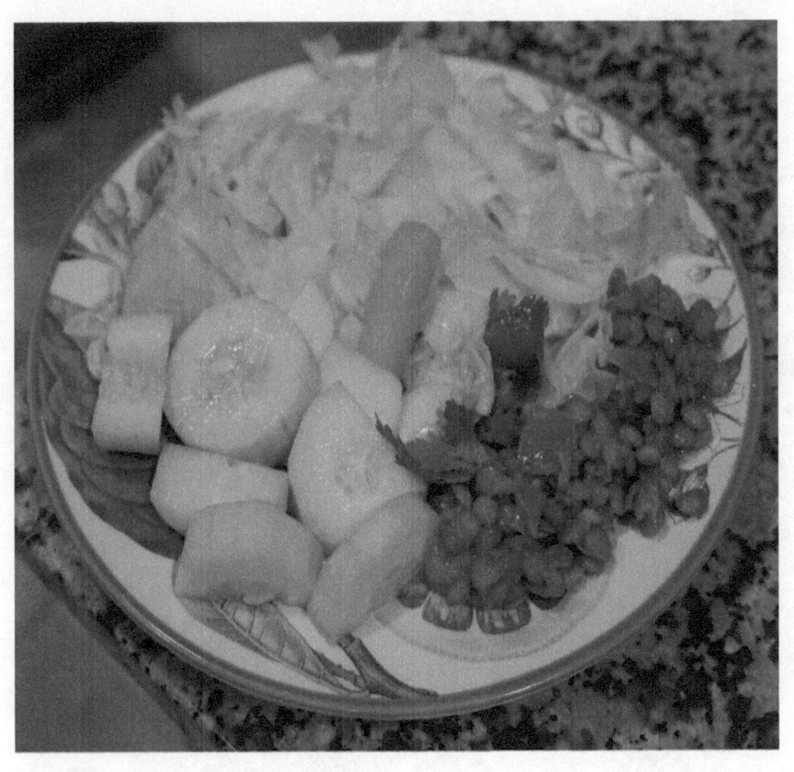

Lentil Green Masoor with salad 2.5 0z
**Cal 90**
**Carbs 10g**
**Fats 0g**
**Protein 10gm**

Ingredients
Tandoori paste grilled chicken
Cucumbers
Lettuce

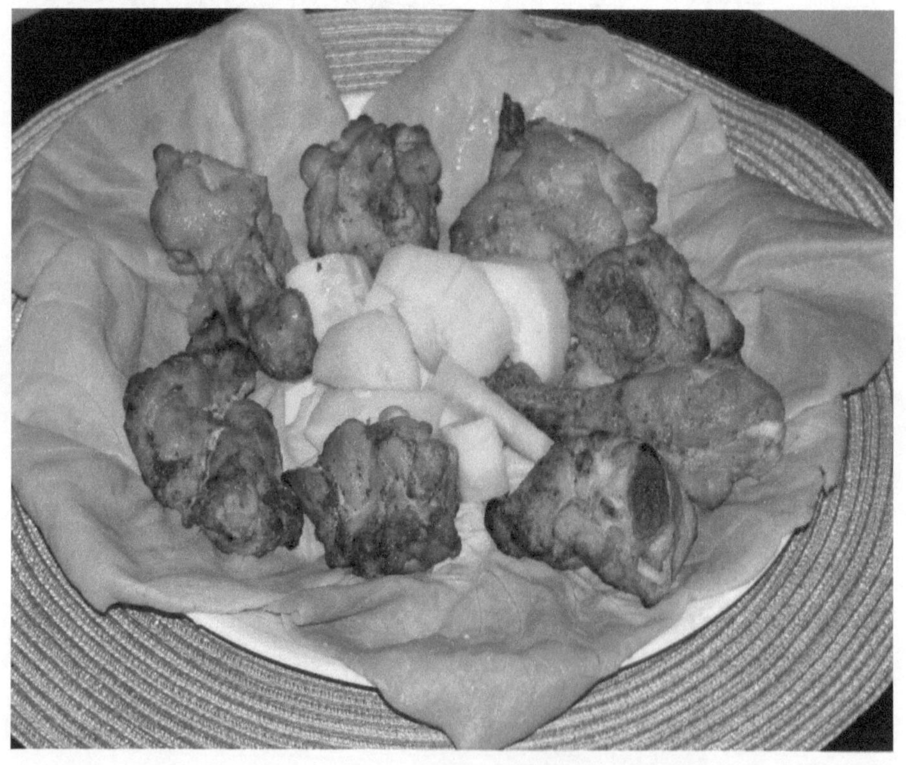

Chicken Tandoori, 4oz, **Cal 152 Carbs
2.6g, Fat 1.9g, Protein 31gm**

Okra with salad Cal 174/cup
**Carbs 14g, fat 6g, protein 2g**

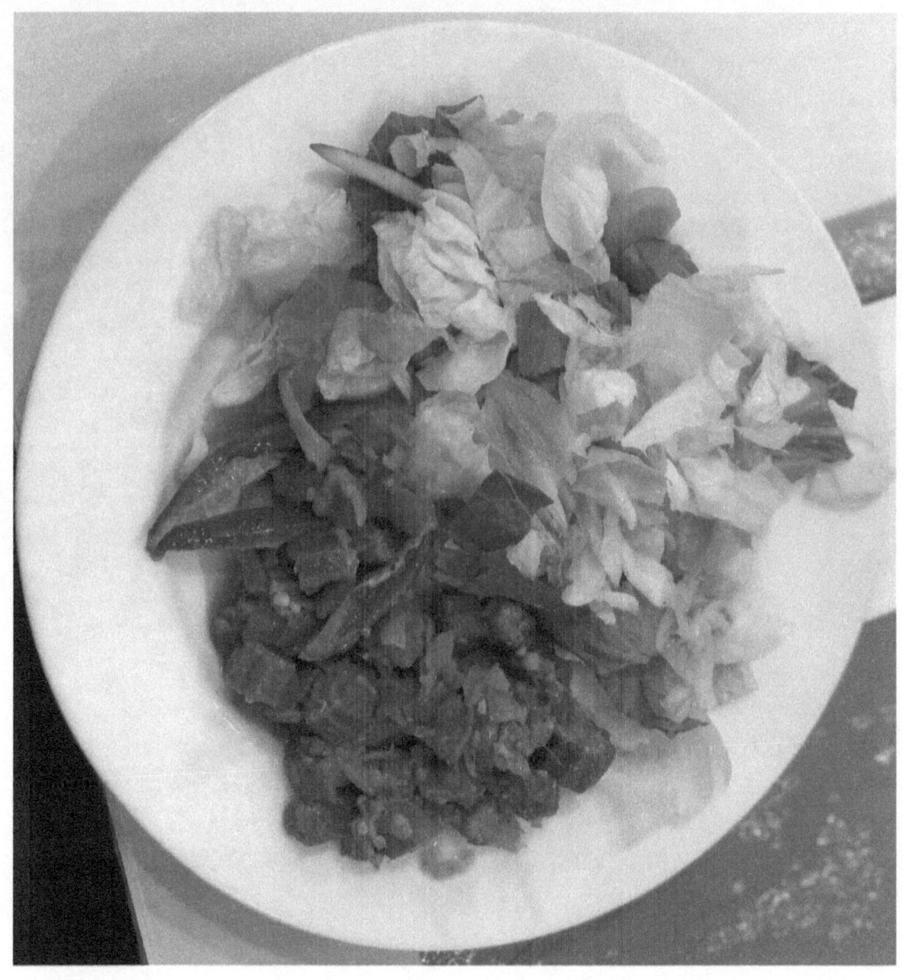

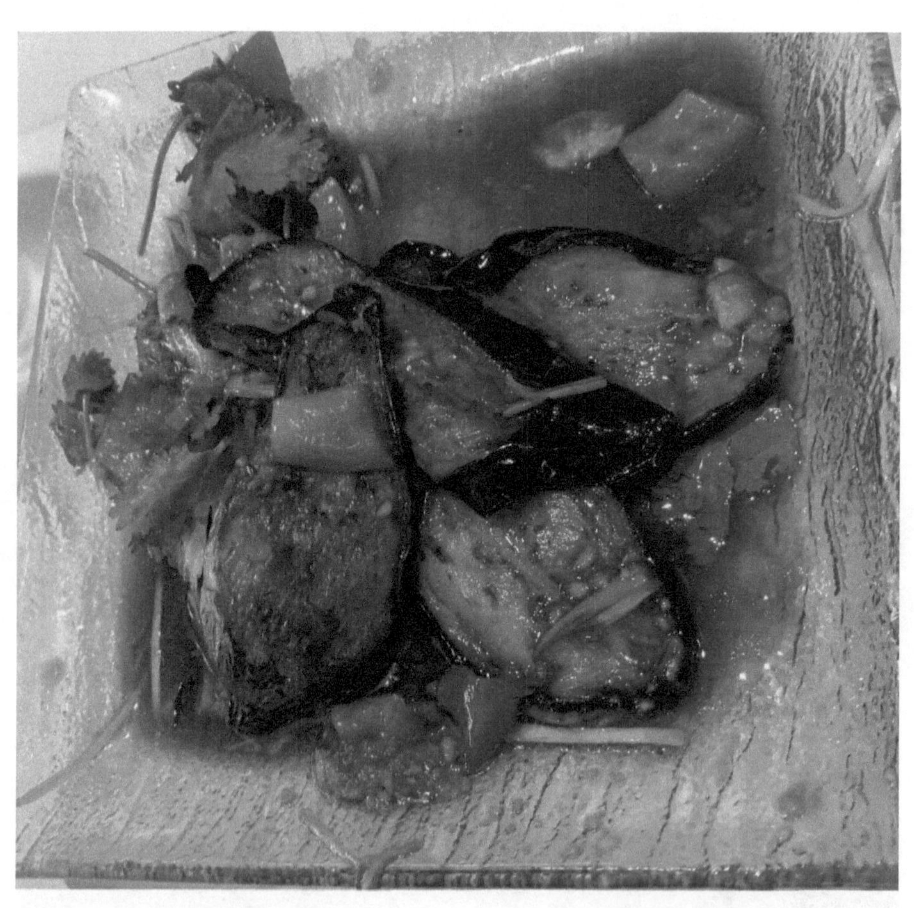

**Egg Plant Salad 100g per 118 cals
26.6 g carbs, 0.6g fat, 4.4g Protein**

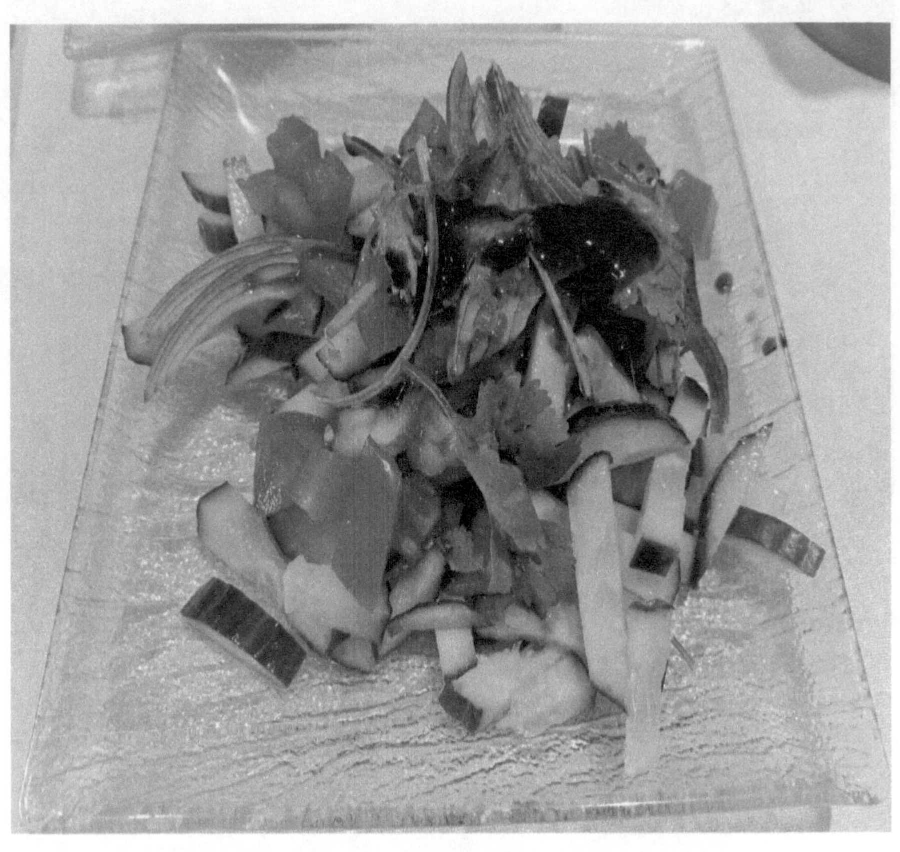

**Cucumber Salad with Dressing**
**75 Cals for 1 bowl**
**8g carbs, 3g fat, 2g protein**

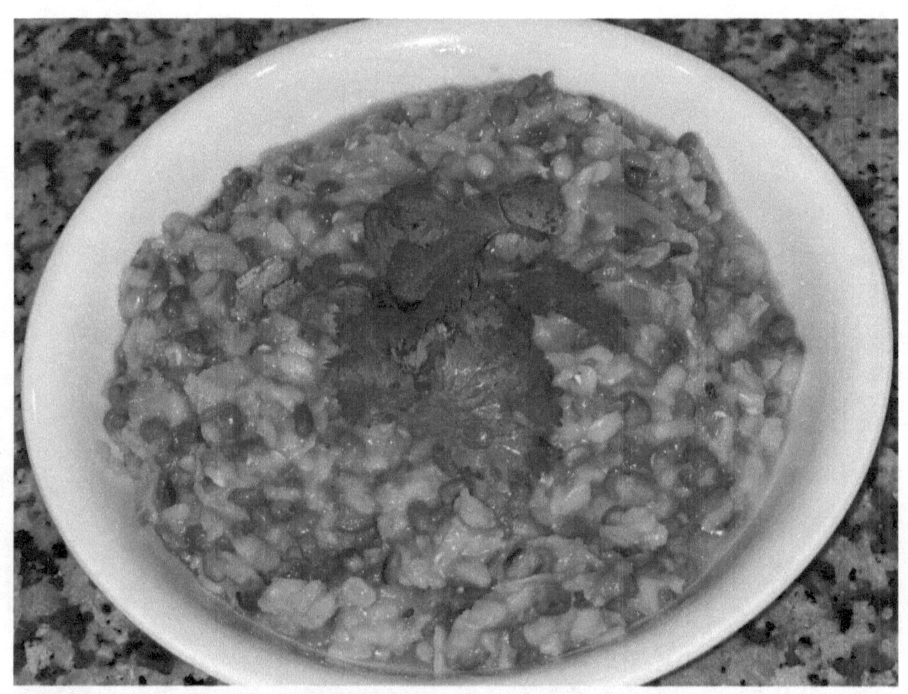

**Moong Dal cooked 1 cup**
**212 cal, 40gm carbs, 0.8g fat, 15g Prot**

**Grilled Pomfret 320gm
Cals 224, carbs none, fat 10g,
Protein 30g**

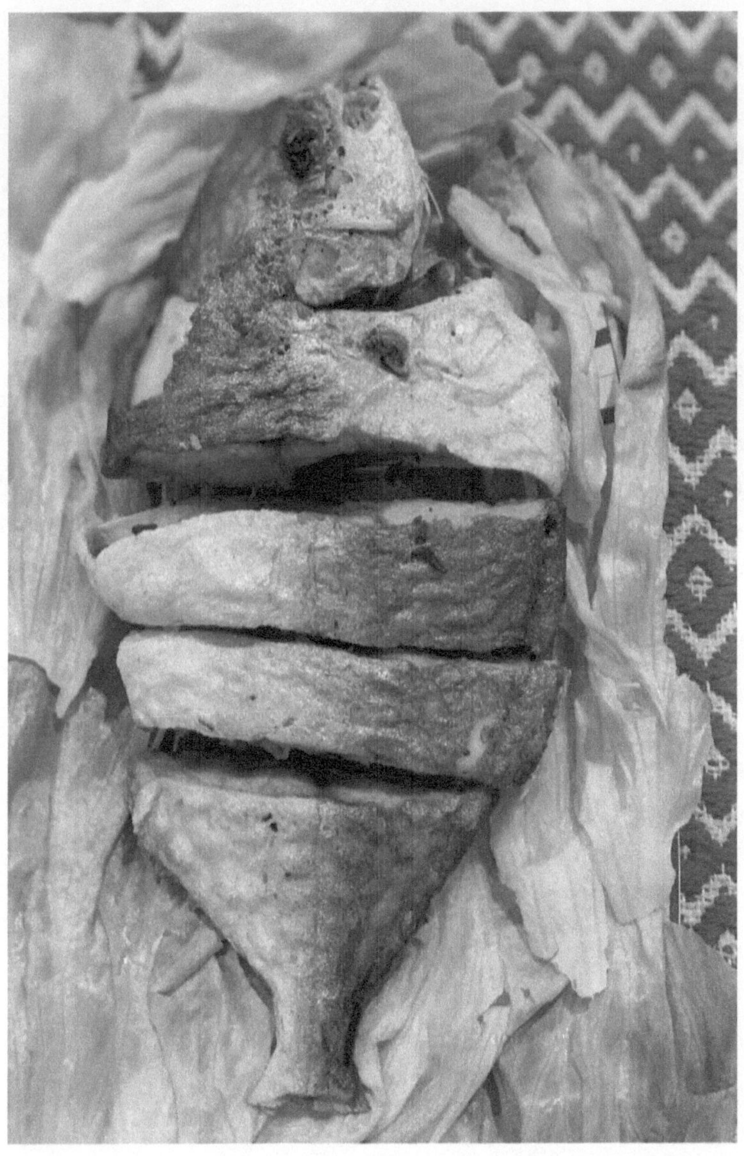

## Fast food Cheat Sheet

1. I eat fast food every day, but never gain weight. You just need to know what to eat.
2. Skip dressings, mayo, and replace ketchup with hot sauce.
3. Lime/Lemon for dressing.
4. No fried food, only grilled.
5. No bread, pasta, rice, croutons.
6. If salad calories are over 200 it is not salad, pay attention to the hidden calories.

## Processed foods

Unfortunately, the food industry is still misleading people. They are adding a lot of fructose syrup as well as additive and chemicals for the food which unfortunately can be a significant factor in weight gain. I think if you look for food which is organic and without any additives, maybe it would be healthy, although I never tried it myself often enough. Instead my recommendation would be to keep it simple and just go back to basics again and then gradually introduce processed food as tolerated

## Supplements

Role of Vitamins/minerals/Water

A lot of people ask me about vitamins and should they start to take multivitamins and minerals. My advice is simple, please check your levels and take vitamins if needed. Unfortunately, people tend to eat more of these than they really need, and consumption of vitamins and supplements is too high. Of course, if you have low levels you will need to take extra, especially the important minerals such as potassium sodium chromium zinc and selenium, along with fat soluble vitamins such as ADEK, water soluble B12 and folate as well as Vitamin C. Iron is also important. Vitamins are the building blocks of our bodies, so it is important to maintain the right amount, and you should pay special attention to potassium and magnesium levels, because they are helpful with muscle cramps and for restless leg syndrome

Water is important for those on any diet, maintaining water levels to make sure adequate hydration is essential, especially if you are on a Ketogenic diet.

Drink before you eat and drink enough water throughout day. I used a lot of Splenda, and I will tell you I know dietitians don't like that, but I don't see a problem with it myself.

Soda.

My advice about soda is that I have personally drink lot of sodas, so I was not against them, but they must be diet sodas in moderation. This also applies to coffee, which is one of my weaknesses. I tend to drink a lot of coffee and tea. A good alternative is green tea, which is pretty loaded with good nutrients.

**Frequently asked questions**

1. Constipation: You may encounter a lot of constipation issues because your water intake is increased and veggies use a lot of water to digest. Caffeinated drinks, such as hot coffee can help address these kinds of problems.

2. Hair loss: I did not have it. I haven't heard about weight loss issues causing hair loss, but ensure you have the right Vitamin D levels to avoid any problems.

3. Fatigue: Staying hydrated is important to avoid fatigue problems, caffeine drinks can also help, and

here is an area when taking extra vitamins or minerals can make a difference, so keep a check on your levels.

4. Flu symptoms: It has been mentioned that if you try a ketogenic diet, initially you might encounter flulike symptoms. It didn't happen to me, but I believe if you go slowly on the diet you can avoid those symptoms.

5. Deficiency: You can have a deficiency of minerals and vitamins, like magnesium. I didn't realize that water soluble vitamin deficiency folates very quickly, so make sure to take vitamin C and folic acid to avoid deficiency and you can also take Vitamin D.

6. Transition to a new diet: I think that you have to realize that you're going to have a new lifestyle, so this would be more appropriate saying it is a transition to new life. Adjusting to it all, such as what to do with the percentage of carbohydrate and I would suggest that you change gradually. Instead of changing a percent every month, just check your weight and if it goes up make sure you cut down on the carbohydrates again until the weight goes. But I would still avoid simple carbohydrates once at your weight, and stick to complex carbohydrates

and the basic principle of portion control.

## Brain Gut Axis

Our intestines are lined with neurons. These cells do not only regulate the activities of the intestine, but they also give feedback to the brain. The composition of the intestinal microbiota shows a dynamic equilibrium in a healthy condition. The microbiota's delicate balance is essential for health because dysbacteriosis, a microbial imbalance, increases the host's susceptibility to disease.

Within this axis, the gut microbiota affects brain function through 3 pathways that produce a bidirectional flow of information. The first of these is the immunoregulatory pathway, in which the microbiota interact with immune cells in such a way as to affect the levels of cytokines, cytokinetic reaction factor, and prostaglandin. As a result, brain function is affected. The second is the neuroendocrine pathway. The gut microbiome may affect the hypothalamic-pituitary-adrenal (HPA) axis and the central nervous system (CNS) by regulating the secretion of neurotransmitters such as cortisol, tryptophan, and serotonin (5-HT). The third is the vagus nerve pathway, in which the enteric nervous system plays an important role.

Not to bore you with all the terms and pathway, but the information to take from this is that a lot of people don't know, but if there's a problem with these bacteria, then it can lead to not only sleep problems but also weight gain, and even in a lot of other issues. One example is in shift work disorder, where people have varied shifts. These are also disturbed.

## Long Term Effects

I am not aware of any deaths from the ketogenic diet. Adverse effects are common. Limitations like any diet.

## Summary

- **Lifestyle change! Simple. Net calories matter**
- **Asses your calories intake at present. Don't use 2000 calories guideline.**
- **Refer to page on CALCULATIONS**
- **Define your goals like if you want to lose 1lb in 1 week or 2 weeks which means 3500 calories less over 1 week or 2 weeks.**
- **Go slow and steady.**
- **Optimize sleep. Get sleep evaluation if needed.**
- **Remember to cut down carbs to ¼ or less total intake especially refined ones as carbs make you hungrier. Proteins and green veggies help satiety.**

- **Take multivitamins and supplements, water. Check levels if needed.**
- **Try to walk at least 30 minutes daily**
- **Meditate, appreciate life, remember more you follow easier it becomes.**
- **Harder battle is to keep it same.**

## Journey Continues

My journey and struggle continue as I am able to keep my weight reduced and help lot of my family members, friends, patients and readers.

Please visit website www.dietsleepexercise.org, www.lifestyletvchannel.com
Facebook lifestyleTV USA
Youtube Lifestyle TV USA - YouTube
Twitter dietsleepexercise@mubasher009
Instagram https://www.instagram.com/lifestyletvusa

Follow podcast, chat, social media for updated information

I would love to hear individual success stories as we keep on learning more every day.

## Bibliography


1. Wikipedia Ketogenic diet www.wikipedia.com
2. International Classification of Sleep disorders ICD3, 3rd edition
3. NIH/weight Control nih.gov
4. Myfitness pal calories www.myfitnesspal.com
5. Paul Kenny, Scientific American: Is Obesity an addiction Sep 01, 2013
6. Rexford Ahima MD, Antwi, Endo Metab Clin North Am. 2008 Dec, 37(4):811-823

## About the Author

**Mubasher Fazal MD (Dr. Mobi)** is a Board-Certified Sleep specialist practicing in the US. He finished medical school in Pakistan, and was awarded with the silver medal for Academic excellence. He has been honored to serve the VA and DOD. With over 22 years' experience in the private sector, he has a special interest in the relationship between sleep and weight. He has served as Head of Medicine and Associate Program Director for Physician Assistant program. Currently, is now Medical Director of Sleep Clinic.

He has famous TV show as Lifestyle with Dr. Mobi, Podcaster recognized as one of Top podcaster Worldwide. He was Keynote speaker for major events, Celebrity recognized worldwide won over 14 Awards including Telly Awards 2021.Check out at Lifestyle TV USA on YouTube, social media Facebook as well as Instagram.

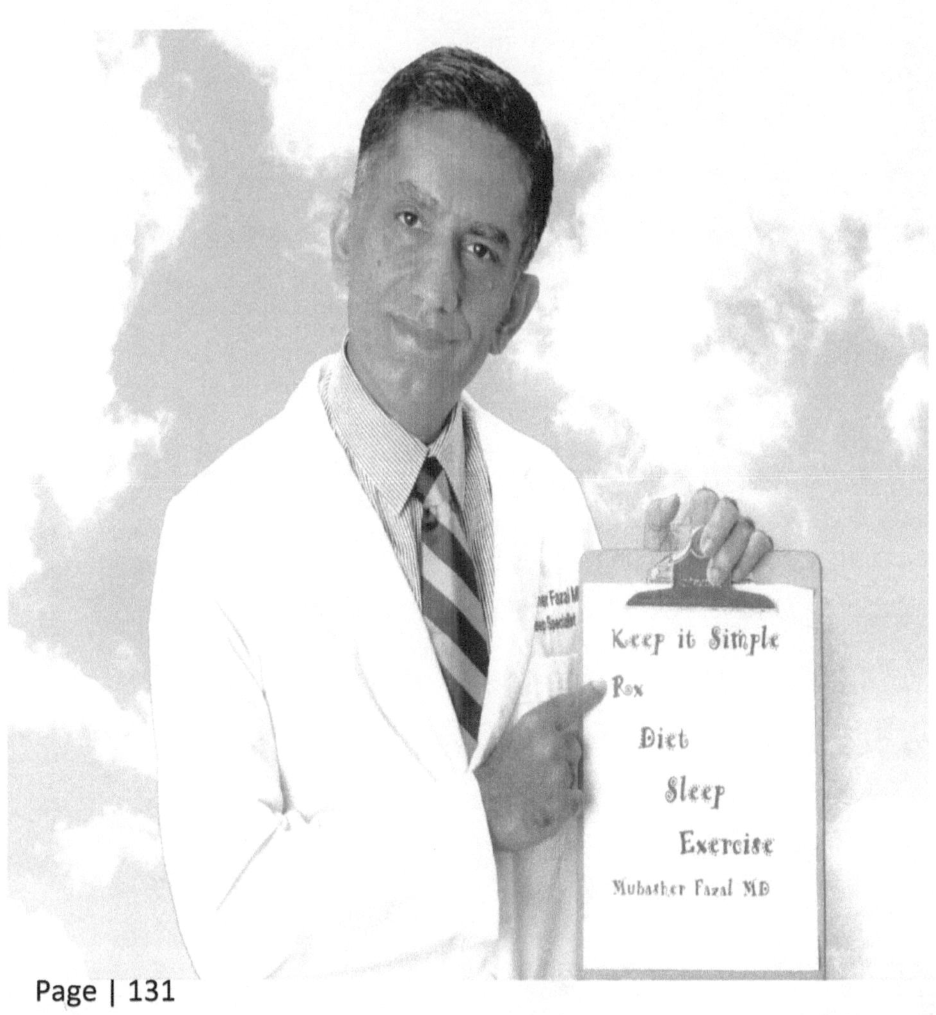

www.ingramcontent.com/pod-product-compliance
Lightning Source LLC
Chambersburg PA
CBHW031127250726
48655CB00002B/549